PARENT/CAREGIVER SUPPORT OF CHILDREN'S *Playfulness* (PC-SCP)

Amiya Waldman-Levi, PhD, OTR/L, and **Anita Bundy,** ScD, OT/L, FAOTA, FOTARA

AOTA American Occupational Therapy Association

AOTA Vision 2025
As an inclusive profession, occupational therapy maximizes health, well-being, and quality of life for all people, populations, and communities through effective solutions that facilitate participation in everyday living.

Mission Statement
The American Occupational Therapy Association advances occupational therapy practice, education, and research through standard-setting and advocacy on behalf of its members, the profession, and the public.

AOTA Staff
Sherry Keramidas, *Executive Director*
Matthew Clark, *Chief Officer, Innovation & Engagement*

Elizabeth Dooley, *Vice President, Strategic Marketing & Communications*
Laura Collins, *Director of Communications and Publications*
Ashley Hofmann, *Acquisitions & Development Manager, AOTA Press*
Amy Ricci, *Product Manager & Business Analyst, AOTA Press*

Rebecca Rutberg, *Director, Marketing*
Amanda Goldman, *Marketing Manager*
Jennifer Folden, *Brand Designer*

American Occupational Therapy Association, Inc.
6116 Executive Boulevard, Suite 200
North Bethesda, MD 20852-4929
www.aota.org
To order: 1-800-729-AOTA (2682) or store.aota.org

ISBN: 978-1-56900-635-1
eBOOK ISBN: 978-1-56900-636-8
Library of Congress Control Number: 2023938443

Cover design by Steve Parrish, AOTA, North Bethesda, MD
Composition by Manila Typesetting Company, Manila, Philippines
Printed by Gasch Printing, Odenton, MD

Suggested citation: Waldman-Levi, A., & Bundy, A. (2023). *Parent/Caregiver Support of Children's Playfulness (PC–SCP)*. AOTA Press.

Contents

*Electronic versions of these forms are available online for clinical use. Readers who purchased this assessment directly from AOTA will automatically see this content on their AOTA Digital Library bookshelf at https://library.aota.org. Readers who purchased this book through a different vendor should contact customerservice@aota.org or call 800-729-2682 to set up a Digital Library bookshelf and access the electronic forms.

Acknowledgments

As clinicians, researchers, and play partners, we believe in the power of play and being playful for family and child health and wellness. Societal, cultural, economic, and health issues influence children's play and playfulness and the support parents or caregivers provide to its development. The Parent/Caregiver Support of Children's Playfulness (PC–SCP) assessment is the product of years of work with parents and children, observing and analyzing the essence of joint play experiences. We hope that the PC–SCP will serve pediatric clinicians in observing joint play experiences to guide them in clinical decision making to support children's and families' health and well-being.

We express our deepest gratitude to several individuals whose contributions have been instrumental to the development of the PC–SCP assessment and manual.

Mindy Garfinkel, OTD, OTR/L, ATP, is a clinical associate professor of occupational therapy at Yeshiva University in New York. She received her OTD from Quinnipiac University and her master's from New York University. She has more than 30 years of clinical experience, primarily in pediatrics and school-based practice. Dr. Garfinkel has served on several national committees, published, contributed to continuing education products, and developed materials for advanced certification in school-based practice. Dr. Garfinkel authored Chapter 6, "Use of the PC–SCP in School Settings," drawing on her vast experience in a school-based setting providing direct and indirect support and coaching teachers and other stakeholders in facilitating student success.

Patricia Grady-Dominguez, PhD, OTR/L, is an adjunct assistant professor and postdoctoral scholar in the Department of Occupational Therapy at Colorado State University in Fort Collins. Dr. Grady-Dominguez completed her PhD at Colorado State University in 2022. She performed the Rasch analyses of PC–SCP data, created the key form, and offered invaluable insights into the findings.

Amber N. Cope, MA, is a clinical psychology doctoral candidate at Long Island University in Brooklyn, New York. Ms. Cope assisted in scoring numerous parent–child joint play recordings and contributed to the refinement of the PC–SCP scoring criteria.

Piermiline Datilus, an occupational therapy doctorate student at Katz School of Science and Health, Yeshiva University, assisted in writing case descriptions. We are grateful to the families who let us learn about their joint play experiences. These observations gave life to this coding scheme. Last, but not least, we thank our former students from Mercy College, Long Island University, and Yeshiva University who assisted in data collection, scoring, and transcribing observations.

About the Authors

Amiya Waldman-Levi, PhD, OTR/L, has more than 20 years of experience in occupational therapy practice, research, and education. Dr. Waldman-Levi's research agenda focuses on promoting individuals', families', and caregivers' resiliency to overcome the impact of adversity on their social–emotional functioning. She has published widely on topics related to parent–child relationships, adversity, and cognition. Dr. Waldman-Levi is the director of scholarship and research at the occupational therapy doctorate program at Katz School of Science and Health at Yeshiva University in New York. She holds BSc, MSc, and PhD degrees from the Hebrew University of Jerusalem. Dr. Waldman-Levi has completed postdoctoral training at the Center for Attachment Research at the New School for Social Research and additional postdoctoral training in assessment and intervention with adults with significant cognitive and executive deficits at Mercy College in Dobbs Ferry, New York.

Anita Bundy, ScD, OT/L, FAOTA, FOTARA, has more than 40 years experience in occupational therapy practice, research, and education. Dr. Bundy focuses her research on promoting and understanding play across the lifespan and on measurement development. She has taught play theory and assessment to occupational therapists and other professionals working with children on five continents. Dr. Bundy is professor and chair of the Department of Occupational Therapy at Colorado State University in Fort Collins. She also has an appointment in the Faculty of Medicine and Health at the University of Sydney, Sydney, New South Wales, Australia. She holds a BS degree from Western Michigan University in Kalamazoo and an MS and ScD from Boston University. She did postdoctoral work at Northwestern University in Chicago.

1

Introduction to the Parent/Caregiver Support of Children's Playfulness

Play, children's main occupation, is essential to growth and development (American Occupational Therapy Association [AOTA], 2008; Skard & Bundy, 2008; Waldman-Levi & Bundy, 2016). Engagement in play contributes to social, emotional, and mental health and allows children to express themselves and endure challenges in restrictive situations (Graber et al., 2021). The United Nations Convention on the Rights of the Child (1989, Article 31) recognizes children's play as both a right and a contributor to development and well-being. Parent–child play is important for enhancing relationships and promoting children's cognitive, social, emotional, and linguistic skills (Waldman-Levi & Bundy, 2016; Waldman-Levi, Finzi-Dottan, & Cope, 2019; Waldman-Levi, Grinion, & Olson, 2019). Ample research supports the importance of adult caregivers in promoting children's play (e.g., Bristow & Atkinson, 2020; Butcher & Gersch, 2014) and playfulness (Waldman-Levi, Finzi-Dottan, & Cope, 2019; Waldman-Levi, Grinion, & Olson, 2019). Also, parent–child play promotes parental as well as child well-being (Román-Oyola et al., 2022). Nonetheless, parent–child engagement in play depends on factors such as lifetime events, child or parental illness or disability, and parental beliefs (Bristow & Atkinson, 2020; Román-Oyola et al., 2022; Waldman-Levi, Finzi-Dottan, & Cope, 2019; Waldman-Levi, Grinion, & Olson, 2019).

When play is the subject of occupational therapy literature, it generally refers to children and the benefits sought through playing. Parent- or caregiver–child play has received less scholarly attention, perhaps because there are so few assessments to evaluate how parents and caregivers support children's playfulness.

Purpose and Scope

The Parent/Caregiver Support of Children's Playfulness (PC–SCP) is an observational tool designed to assess parents' or other caregivers' support of children's playfulness. The PC–SCP is administered while the clinician observes a 15-minute unstructured play session between a parent or caregiver and a child. This clinician-rated instrument can be administered in person, watching a video-recorded session, or via telehealth. The testing environment can be a clinic, school, home, or other environment in which the parent or caregiver and child are comfortable; the testing environment is ideally one familiar to the adult and child and one in which they have played previously. Using the PC–SCP to assess how parents or caregivers support children's playfulness can guide clinicians in developing family-centered interventions. An intervention plan that stems from PC–SCP results can promote parent- or caregiver–child relationships as well as skill development (Waldman-Levi & Bundy, 2016; Waldman-Levi, Bundy, & Shai, 2022).

Target Population and Audience

The PC–SCP targets parents or caregivers of children ages 12 months to 11 years. A *caregiver* is any adult with a primary relationship to the child (e.g., grandparents, teachers, and educational staff members). Populations at risk, such as parents or caregivers who were exposed to adverse life experiences (e.g., trauma, domestic violence, illness) and children experiencing developmental challenges, can benefit from improving joint play and related skills (e.g., social–emotional, cognitive, and communication skills). Pediatric clinicians, including occupational therapists, social workers, psychologists, or speech–language pathologists, may use the PC–SCP.

Educational Training

In addition to providing an avenue for family-centered interventions, the PC–SCP may be useful in educating students or inexperienced practitioners as they play with a child. The resulting analysis could serve as the basis for supervision and enhancing the promotion of therapeutic play (see also Chapters 3, 4, and 5 for information on how to administer the PC–SCP, how to score, and how to interpret scoring). This information can be useful in guiding students and clinicians in making meaning and developing interventions that target PC–SCP findings.

Play and Child Development

Play is an activity in which children are engaged solely because they want to do the activity. Play takes many forms: social, imaginary, gross motor, board games, and so forth (Parham & Primeau, 2008). *Playfulness,* a concept closely related to play, is defined as the "disposition to play" (Skard & Bundy, 2008, p. 71). Unsurprisingly, playfulness is associated with many of the same benefits as play: emotional regulation, creativity, higher cognitive processing, adaptability, and coping (Bergen & Fromberg, 2009; Hess & Bundy, 2003; Saunders et al., 1999). Although playfulness is commonly seen in the context of play, it can also be seen in other activities (e.g., work, chores).

Occupational therapists and other practitioners working with children and families must understand what is expected of children of varying ages as they play (Case-Smith & Kuhaneck, 2008) as well as what motivates children to engage in play activities and be playful. Howard et al. (2017) found that children's positive perceptions of play were associated with usual play activities and playmates. Starting in the preschool years, children develop preferences for playing with certain playmates over others (Hwang & Markson, 2020).

Researchers (e.g., Pontes et al., 2016) often find that children's play preferences differ depending on gender. Boys tend to prefer physical activities (e.g., soccer, climbing trees) and video games, and girls tend to prefer creative activities. Children's play preferences also change with age, with children ages 9 to 13 years more often involved in organized outdoor group activities and children ages 14 to 18 years preferring solitary activities (Auhuber et al., 2019; Imms et al., 2016). Some researchers (Jago et al., 2018; Oberle et al., 2019) have found that children's play preferences are set by age 6 years and maintained through adolescence. Others (Corder et al., 2013; Lam & McHale, 2015; Zahl et al., 2017) have found changes in preferences from middle childhood to adolescence, noticing increased physical activities in early middle childhood (ages 6–8 years) but decreased active play and increased sedentary activity by ages 10 to 12 years.

Perhaps unsurprisingly, some researchers (Auhuber et al., 2019; Männikkö et al., 2020) have found that children who are less engaged in physical play spend more time on screens (e.g., phone, tablet, television, computer). In a recent study conducted in Turkey on computer game playing, mothers reported that their children spent most of their time playing computer games, preferring to stay home and play alone rather than spending time outdoors with peers (Mertol-Ilgar & Cigdem-Karakurt, 2018).

Parent– or Caregiver–Child Play

In joint play, players share physical space and objects, ideas, intentions, and emotions (Pickens & Pizur-Barnekow, 2009; Waldman-Levi & Bundy, 2016; Waldman-Levi, Finzi-Dottan, & Cope, 2019). The adult's role in joint play is to support the child's engagement, exploration, and enjoyment. However, it is important that the adult is also playing.

Children are sensitive to whether their adult playmate is truly playing. If the adult is not playing, it is unlikely that the child will be playing.

An adult's responses in joint play reflect their capacity to identify and interpret the child's behavior and needs (Borelli et al., 2017; Slade, 2007). During joint play, the adult demonstrates support by incorporating a playful attitude, modifying play activities, and flexibly using play materials to capture the child's interests and needs (Waldman-Levi & Bundy, 2016; Waldman-Levi, Finzi-Dottan, & Cope, 2019; Waldman-Levi, Grinion, & Olson, 2019).

Children's growth and development are influenced by their relationships with parents and other adult caregivers (e.g., Fonagy & Target, 1998; Shaver et al., 2010; Slade, 2007). Parent–child play provides parents with an opportunity to witness their child's inner world and for the child to be seen, heard, and understood by a parent (Desmarais, 2006). Maternal behaviors affect children's self-regulation, self-reflection, and sense of independence (Bekar et al., 2015; Borelli et al., 2017; Slade, 2007). Maternal caregiving and a reflective disposition assist mothers to support their child's engagement in challenging tasks (Waldman-Levi, Finzi-Dottan, & Cope, 2019). In a mixed-methods study of maternal caregiving behaviors and joint play during middle childhood, Waldman-Levi, Finzi-Dottan, and Cope (2019) found that mothers with fewer anxious and avoidant caregiving behaviors demonstrated greater support of their children's playfulness. Mothers who were supportive of their children's playfulness allowed their children to take the lead in play and created a safe environment in which children could make errors and figure out solutions. Mothers used joint play time to foster attuned conversations with their child about their social life (Waldman-Levi, Finzi-Dottan, & Cope, 2019).

Studies of paternal behaviors with young children reveal that fathers' support differs from mothers' but is equally as important to children's social–emotional development (Waldman-Levi, 2022). Continued engagement in joint play from infancy onward is essential to building cognitive and social–emotional abilities and playfulness (Howard et al., 2017; Keren et al., 2005; Lindsey & Mize, 2000; Waldman-Levi, Cope, & Olson, 2022). Early signs of mismatch or lack of support during joint play can be addressed through family-centered interventions. Strategies to support parents' or caregivers' play interactions with their child can assist them in building relationships and reducing family conflicts.

Social Isolation and Play

Play is essential to health, development, and learning. Living under severe social restrictions affects play and, thus, may compromise development and health. In a rapid review of 15 studies, Graber et al. (2021) collated evidence on the impact of social isolation on children's play and the extent to which play mitigated adverse effects of quarantine or social isolation on children's health and educational outcomes. Studies were conducted in several environments (i.e., hospitals, juvenile and immigration detention centers, and a refugee camp) and involved various play and leisure activities (i.e., sandbox play, puppetry, toy play, rule-based games, art, reading and writing, music). Graber et al. (2021) noted that restrictions affected children's access to, and frequency of, engagement in play.

The SARS-CoV-2 virus (COVID-19) pandemic and related social restrictions also caused disruptions to play engagement, including where, when, how, and with whom play occurred. In a qualitative study, Pascal and Bertram (2021) explored the experiences of young children during the pandemic. Their thematic analysis of play narratives revealed children's desire to regain their daily life and routines, be with their friends, have extended time to play, and spend time outdoors. Parents reported that their children incorporated COVID-19 pandemic experiences into their play, seemingly in an attempt to make sense of them. In another study of the implications of social isolation during the COVID-19 pandemic with Brazilian families of children younger than age 13 years, Sá et al. (2020) found that, before social isolation, 67.8% of children engaged in physical activities or play at least twice a week; however, during the pandemic, screen time increased significantly.

Play Interaction Across Settings and Diagnostic Populations

Disability influences both type and quality of play (Waldman-Levi, 2022), and the range of activities in which children with disabilities engage is associated with their level of independence (Sanches-Ferreira et al., 2019). Performance skills deficits challenge a child's ability to play, and they affect parent–child play (Gale & Schick, 2008; Graham et al., 2015; Lifter et al., 2011). Researchers have found that children with disabilities participate in solitary play in constrained spaces at school more frequently than children without disabilities. They also tend to participate in less diverse activities than children without disabilities (Sanches-Ferreira et al., 2019). Several authors (e.g., Childress, 2010; De Falco et al., 2010) have reported that children with disabilities gained more benefits from playing with a parent than from playing alone, and the benefits varied depending on which parent was playing with the child. De Falco et al. (2010) found that when children played with their father, they demonstrated more symbolic play than when they played with their mother. The authors surmised that fathers had a decreased tendency to overdemonstrate symbolic play, which may have indirectly encouraged the children to play their own role.

Play is a right for all children and fundamental for their growth, development, and health. Through play, children develop social, emotional, physical, and cognitive skills that contribute to physical and mental health as well as school readiness. Through play with adults, children form strong bonds. The contexts of where children play, and with whom, greatly affect children's play development. Their early play with adult caretakers significantly shapes their social–emotional and cognitive development and translates to how they interact with others. For example, see 7-year-old Molly Wright's (2021) TED Talk, "How Every Child Can Thrive by Five," as she describes the benefits of peek-a-boo and other child–adult play to the developing brain.

2

Conceptual Framework

Co-occupation is an important piece of the Parent/Caregiver Support of Children's Playfulness's (PC–SCP's) theoretical foundation. The PC–SCP is grounded in the concept of co-occupation and assesses how parents or caregivers support their child's playfulness during joint play.

Co-Occupation

Occupational science advocates for the study of human occupations to inform practice with a body of knowledge that promotes health, growth, development, and wellness (Pierce, 2014). In the early days of occupational science, Pierce (2009) coined the term *co-occupation,* which emerged from the interdisciplinary play literature as well as from occupational scientists' interest in the interactive social dimension of occupation, especially that of mothers and children. *Co-occupation* refers to people's engagement in an activity while sharing space, physical features, intention, and emotional states with others (Pickens & Pizur-Barnekow, 2009; Whitcomb, 2012). In this shared experience, the co-occupants influence one another's actions, mental states, and emotions (Waldman-Levi, Grinion, & Olson, 2019). In joint play, a parent's or caregiver's and child's occupations are relational (Scoggin, 1999; Sethi, 2020), influencing and depending on one another. An interruption in the co-occupation of joint play is often manifested in a lack of flow or synchrony (Sethi, 2000; Waldman-Levi, Finzi-Dottan, & Cope, 2019).

Child Playfulness

The PC–SCP is based on the theoretical Model of Playfulness (Bundy & Du Toit, 2014; Skard & Bundy, 2008), which postulates that playfulness reflects a continuum of behaviors ranging from nonplayful to playful and consists of four essential elements:

1. *Intrinsic motivation:* the ability to engage in self-chosen and meaningful play activities
2. *Internal locus of control:* the ability to change play to create more fun and challenge
3. *Freedom from unnecessary constraints of reality:* the ability to determine how close to objective reality a play transaction will be
4. *Framing:* the ability to provide and read social cues (verbal and nonverbal) that support the continuation of play (e.g., Bundy & Du Toit, 2014; Skard & Bundy, 2008).

In joint play, a child's playfulness is influenced by parent or caregiver behaviors and the support they provide to a child playmate. PC–SCP items reflect the Model of Playfulness and the extent to which an adult uses verbal and nonverbal communication to support and promote a child's play and playfulness.

Adult Playfulness

Playfulness is a multidimensional concept, and an internal disposition toward playfulness includes fun-seeking motivation, uninhibitedness, and spontaneity (Proyer, 2012c; Shen et al., 2014). In the psychology literature, *playfulness* has been defined as "the predisposition to frame a situation in such a way as to provide oneself (and possibly others) with amusement, humor, and/or entertainment" (Barnett, 2007, p. 955). It may seem as though playfulness is a way of thinking and play is the external manifestation of this attitude (Guitard et al., 2005). Barnett (2007) reported that playful adults are active, adventurous, cheerful, energetic, friendly, funny, happy, humorous, impulsive, outgoing, sociable, spontaneous, and unpredictable; these qualities manifest similarly in men and women. In contrast, Proyer (2012b) described the prototypic playful adult as extroverted, open, agreeable, following intrinsic life goals, endorsing a pleasurable and engaged life, and perceiving themselves as genuine.

Playfulness serves an adaptive function for adults as well as children. For instance, Magnuson and Barnett (2013) reported that college students who rated themselves as playful incorporated effective coping skills in stressful situations, such as during exams. They explained that playful individuals have lower levels of perceived stress than less playful counterparts; they more frequently use adaptive, stressor-focused coping strategies and are less likely to use negative, avoidant, and escape-oriented strategies. Proyer (2012a) noted that playfulness has adaptive and flexible qualities, allowing adults to approach activities with the same openness of mind with which a child approaches play: The beginning is known, and a precise end is anticipated, but the nature of its unfolding may vary. Being playful can assist when one is faced with a difficult situation. Playful adults perceive difficult situations as challenges, occasions to learn, and possibilities to increase their competence and skills. Moreover, they do not consider mistakes as a failure but rather as an opportunity to learn and grow (Proyer, 2012c). Relying on attachment theory, Gordon (2014) provided further support for the adaptive function playfulness serves in adults' well-being. Gordon (2014) explained that securely attached infants were more able to explore the environment, play, and be playful. In the absence of developmental trauma, playful children turn into playful adults. Gordon also connected adult playfulness with a sense of well-being and satisfaction in life, explaining that playful adults are adaptive, able to cope with life stressors, and live healthy and satisfying lives.

Development and Joint Play

When playing with their very young infant, parents often attribute meaning to the infant's emotional state. Early parent–child joint play commonly involves sensorimotor exchanges such as playing peek-a-boo or tickling (Keren et al., 2005; Shai & Belsky, 2011). A parent who initiates an exchange during joint play often elicits a positive and joyful response from the child (Keren et al., 2005). When a parent or caregiver repeats exchanges and initiations, the infant learns to anticipate their movement, touch, and facial expression. For example, an infant may burst into laughter by looking at their mother's face when she covers it with her hands, before she even says "peek-a-boo." In an observational study of mother–infant dyads with infants ages 3 to 4 months, Pizur-Barnekow et al. (2014) found that mothers spent the greatest amount of time using attention-supporting rather than attention-directing strategies or controlled play. *Controlled play* refers to when a mother prohibits certain play with an object or uses a toy to get her child's attention. *Attention-directing behaviors* consist of the mother pointing, guiding, or handing her child a toy, and *attention-supporting behaviors* consist of the mother responding to her child's expressed interest in an object or toy, as well as consistent use of facial expressions and eye contact. Attention-supporting strategies promote synchronous interactions and give infants a sense of a supportive presence. Children's symbolic play begins between ages 8 and 15 months, and pretend play begins between ages 2 and 3 years (Fonagy & Target, 1998). In symbolic and pretend joint play, children learn to incorporate representations of objects and actions into play and to represent thoughts and feelings abstractly. If play supports the development of early mental capacity, then joint play is the context in which parents can support their child to develop mental capacity as well as motor, cognitive, linguistic, and social skills.

In middle childhood (ages 6 to 11 or 12 years), play often includes board games, sports, and computer games, all of which can be done with a parent. Such play involves rules and requires various degrees of interaction (Howard et al., 2017; Oren, 2008). When done jointly, these types of play provide opportunities for parents and children to give and respond to cues, overcome obstacles, challenge oneself and others, and be creative and mischievous. Oren (2008) found that board games, in particular, promoted emotional and impulse regulation and provided opportunities to understand rules and relationships.

Factors Affecting Joint Play

Family culture influences the content and frequency of parent–child joint play (Waldman-Levi, 2022; Waldman-Levi & Weintraub 2009). Several studies have shown how mother–child play varies between families of different ethnicities or countries of origin. For instance, mothers and children of American and European origin often engage in child-led and symbolic or make-believe play. In contrast, mothers and children of Asian origin engage in parent-led play and imitation of real-life experiences (Bazyk et al., 2003; Parham & Primeau, 2008).

In recent years, societal and economic changes have shifted family dynamics and practices. The traditional role of fathers as sole or primary breadwinner is no longer the norm. Fathers' role as caregivers has also changed; in some families, fathers are the primary caregivers; in others, parents share child-rearing responsibilities (Cabrera et al., 2014; Jones & Mosher, 2013). A national survey in the United States of 10,403 fathers of children from infancy through age 18 years confirmed this change. The researchers reported differences in fathers' involvement in their children's lives, with fathers who are at home more reporting that they spend more time playing with their children (Jones & Mosher, 2013).

Mothers and fathers differ in the ways in which they play with their children. Several researchers (John et al., 2013; StGeorge et al., 2015) reported that fathers tend to be active and physical when playing with their children. Other researchers described fathers incorporating competitive play and challenges and exhibiting age-mate behaviors (Cabrera & Roggman, 2017; Flanders et al., 2009; Waldman-Levi, Cope, & Olson, 2022). Waldman-Levi (2021) also found that the more frequently fathers displayed playful and supportive behaviors during joint play, the more playful and engaged their child was. Moreover, when fathers displayed an increased quality of support for playful behaviors, their child was more skillful during play.

In contrast to fathers, mothers' play is more structured. Mothers tend to demonstrate empathy as they guide, direct, and teach their children during joint play (John et al., 2013; Waldman-Levi & Weintraub, 2009). Interviewing mothers and fathers after a play experience with their child revealed that the mothers valued play as an activity that allows them to connect with their child and educate them (Waldman-Levi, Finzi-Dottan, & Cope, 2019).

Parent–child play may be especially important for children with disabilities; several studies of dyads of children with disabilities (e.g., Childress, 2010; De Falco et al., 2010) reported that playing with a parent elicited better play abilities than when the child played alone. Unsurprisingly, the benefits may vary on the basis of which parent is playing with the child.

Benefits of Joint Play

Parent or caregiver engagement in joint play can strengthen their relationship with a child and contribute to the development of self-regulation and social skills (Price & Miner Stephenson, 2009; Scoggin, 1999). According to Winnicott (1999), one of the core aspects of mother–child interaction during play is maternal presence, which provides the child with the sense of safety required to play (Waldman-Levi, 2021). In a study grounded in constructivist theory, Sethi (2020) described the mothering role as being relational and consisting of caregiver, nurturer, educator, protector, and learner qualities. This conceptualization of mothering can also be applied to joint play when a parent or caregiver helps the child overcome challenges to continue with the play. Nurturing is observed through the affective tone, care, and praise provided during joint play. The parent or caregiver promotes development by encouraging the child to engage in ability-suited activities as well as teaching, demonstrating, or assisting the child with manipulating and using objects, space, or ideas in play. A parent or caregiver supports their child during play by providing cues or setting boundaries to keep the child secure. Last, joint play is a relational and reciprocal form of co-occupation. Parents' or caregivers' behaviors and thoughts change as they develop greater skills in parenting, caring, educating, and playing with their child.

3

PC–SCP Description and Administration

The Parent/Caregiver Support of Children's Playfulness (PC–SCP) assessment is an observational and behavioral coding system of 15-minute joint play between a parent or caregiver and child. It consists of 16 items rated on the quality of the behavior, ranging from 0 (*low; the parent or caregiver is unaware of child's needs*) to 3 (*high; parent or caregiver response closely matches child ability and preference*). When a behavior is not evident because it is irrelevant to the activity, then a score of *not applicable* (NA) is assigned (Waldman-Levi & Bundy, 2016). When calculating the average score, do not include items with NA scoring because it will lower the scoring. If two items are rated as NA, then the sum of the scored items will be divided by 14 and not 16. Upon completion of the scoring, the examiner can calculate the average score and then compare it with the data from nonclinical samples provided in Chapter 7.

Administration and Scoring Procedures

The PC–SCP reflects an observational paradigm (Brock et al., 2020) in which the dyad is engaged in joint play for an assigned time. The examiner or coder views the observation in its entirety (whether recorded or live) before scoring items (Brock et al., 2020; Fujiwara & Daibo, 2014; Schneiderman et al., 2014). The parent or caregiver and child are invited to play together as they usually do for 15 minutes. When conducting the PC–SCP in an environment that is unfamiliar to the dyad, the examiner should allow about 5 to 10 minutes of free play before assessing the joint play experience.

Observing Joint Play

Observation is the gold standard for assessing parent–child interactions to identify parental or child-related issues, as well as problems within the dyadic relationship (Gridley et al., 2018). The PC–SCP can be scored live or video recorded and then scored. Video recording is commonly used in studies of child development and behavior, parent–child interaction, and parenting (e.g., Gridley et al., 2018; Harvey et al., 2009; McNeil & Repetti, 2021; Sparrman, 2005); live observation is more feasible in clinical settings.

When comparing scoring from live and video-recorded observations, some researchers (Gridley et al., 2018; Sparrman, 2005) have found that both methods provide ecologically valid information and similar results. Moreover, interobserver reliability can be attained using either mode. However, the video mode tends to yield higher levels of interobserver reliability (Gridley et al., 2018).

Cultural and Social Biases

Whether the observation is video recorded and then scored or scored live, observer characteristics may affect scoring (Harvey et al., 2009). For example, some researchers (Harvey et al., 2009; Wang et al., 2007) found differences when raters of a different ethnicity from that of the parent and child they observed scored child defiant or negative behaviors compared with when raters of the same ethnicity as the dyad scored these behaviors. To address cultural or ethnicity-related biases, the examiner should reflect on their scoring, especially when scoring a dyad from a background different from theirs.

Another scoring consideration comes when the parent or child is very aware of being observed, which can affect their behavior. For adults, the feeling of being observed might decrease after about 5 minutes. Children's feelings of being observed generally subside as soon as the parent or caregiver is at ease. At times, children incorporate the feeling of being observed into their play (Sparrman, 2005). To reduce potential negative influences, it is important to explain the reason for recording or taking notes; show the parent or caregiver and child the device (e.g., videorecorder, paper and pencil) and answer any questions they have.

Examiner Training

The PC–SCP is conceptually grounded in occupational science and the occupational therapy literature and designed for use by occupational therapists, but it can also be used by other professionals working with children and families (e.g., psychologists, social workers, speech–language therapists). The examiner should be skilled in observational and behavioral coding as well as in observing joint play in different environments (e.g., indoors, outdoors, school, home). To prepare to administer the PC–SCP, the examiner must practice scoring video-recorded joint play experiences with a trained colleague to develop skills in observing and using this assessment.

PREPARATION

Before using the PC–SCP for clinical or research purposes, examiners should observe children playing in different settings and with different playmates. To gain a broader perspective on joint play and playfulness, it is important to observe typically and atypically developing children as well as children of different ages. Many examiners will benefit from the case descriptions in Chapter 5: reading them, scoring them, comparing their ratings with those provided, and studying the scoring rationale when there are differences. Generally, differences in rating between a 2 and 3 are not problematic because both reflect satisfactory behavior. However, differences in rating between a 1 and 2 may indicate a misinterpretation of the scoring criteria.

After scoring the transcripts in Chapter 5 and reaching a close match with the scoring form provided for each case, examiners should partner with a trained colleague to observe a dyad and compare scores. At this phase of the training, we recommend video recording the dyad and following all guidelines. Each examiner should score the video separately; both examiners can then compare their scores and discuss differences. If needed, they can observe the recording together to resolve differences in scoring. Examiners should repeat the process several times until their scoring reaches 80% agreement. To calculate the level of agreement, count the number of items the two examiners scored the same, then divide that number by the total number of items (16) and multiply by 100. (If there are items that score as NA, then the sum will be divided by the number of scored items.)

For research purposes, we recommend that this process be formalized in multiphase training to achieve reliability in scoring among examiners. In multiphase training, the first two phases are similar to the clinical training described here. In the first phase, examiners thoroughly review the manual and scoring criteria outlined in Chapter 4. In the second phase, examiners read and score the case description in Chapter 5 and review and discuss differences with each other. Researchers then engage in a third training phase, in which they create and score two (or more) videos of children and parents (or other caregivers) who have the same characteristics as the participants they plan to study. Examiners are advised to move to the next phase only after they achieve competency in the current phase. After each examiner scores the first video-recorded joint play experience, they should compare their scoring and discuss any differences. After differences have been resolved, examiners can repeat the process with the second recording. If, after the second round of scoring, there are still significant differences (<80% overall agreement), then the process must be repeated. If examiners reach an acceptable level of agreement, they can proceed with their research plan, separately scoring 20% of their sample on which to calculate and report interrater reliability.

SELF-REFLECTION

Acknowledging that cultural, racial, or other differences may affect scoring of joint play, we recommend that examiners regularly engage in self-reflection. A conversation with the parent or caregiver regarding how they perceive play with their child, what challenges they experience, and the ways in which they deal with those challenges will often assist examiners in understanding behaviors (Waldman-Levi, 2021; Waldman-Levi, Finzi-Dottan, & Cope, 2019; Waldman-Levi, Grinion, & Olson, 2019). Examiners should also privately reflect on their own biases, especially in cases in which scoring is unusually low or high. Consulting with an experienced colleague or mentor is also an excellent strategy.

4

Scoring Guidelines and Interpretation

The Parent/Caregiver Support of Children's Playfulness (PC–SCP) consists of 16 items. Ratings are assigned and interpreted as shown in Table 4.1. In situations in which behavior was not observed because of the type of play the child was performing, rather than because of ability, a score of *not applicable* should be assigned. Table 4.2 shows a blank scoring form; the scoring form is also available in Appendix A.

TABLE 4.1. Scoring Guidelines

Item Description	Rating Scale Description
1. Parent/caregiver is *actively supporting* the child's engagement in free play. Parent/caregiver's support of child's engagement is evident through several behaviors, such as parent or caregiver being seated close to or at a distance from the child; parent's or caregiver's attention, focus, and interest are with the child's play activities. *Note.* With infants (as young as 6 months old) the parent/caregiver may position the infant in varied ways. In scoring, consider how positioning supported the infant's engagement in free play.	**0 (low)**—Parent/caregiver seems clearly nonsupportive of the child's engagement. This may include the following behaviors: Parent/caregiver sits a distance from the child; their attention seems to be shifted away; when the child attempts to attract the parent's or caregiver's attention, they seem reluctant or disinterested. **1 (mild)**—Parent/caregiver's supportive engagement is less than optimal. They are not focused on the child's needs in play. **2 (moderate)**—Parent/caregiver seems to actively support the child's engagement in free play. However, the parent/caregiver may occasionally miss a few of the play activities or interactions occurring during the free-play session. **3 (high)**—Parent/caregiver presence is supportive of the child's engagement. The activities or interactions are important to them. Parent's/caregiver's attention might drift, but that occurs rarely, and the parent/caregiver effortlessly reengages with the child's play.

(Continued)

TABLE 4.1. Scoring Guidelines *(Cont.)*

Item Description	Rating Scale Description
2. Parent/caregiver supports the child's engagement in the activity *for the process* rather than primarily for the end product (building, assembling, and "getting the job done"). *Note.* The child may be interested in the outcome as well as the process (e.g., in playing a game, the child would like to win), but the outcome is not the most important thing, and the parent/caregiver captures that. The child would like to keep playing regardless of the outcome.	**0 (low)**—Parent/caregiver is not supportive of the child's engagement in the activity or the process. **1 (mild)**—Parent/caregiver is entirely concentrated on the child completing play activities. Their prompts give the impression that each play activity is a task that needs to be completed; the atmosphere is "getting the job done," or the parent/caregiver primarily seeks to teach the child. **2 (moderate)**—Parent/caregiver shows clear support of the child's engagement in both the process and the outcome. Although they may direct the child to achieve the outcome, at other times the parent/caregiver encourages the child to engage in the process. It seems as though the parent's/caregiver's support is balanced between process and outcome. **3 (high)**—Parent/caregiver is supportive of the child's engagement in the activity for the process, as the child perceives it. It does not seem as though the outcome is more important than the process. The prompts and encouragement they give the child focus on the process rather than on the outcome.
3. Parent/caregiver *helps* the child *overcome barriers or obstacles* to persist with the activity. When scoring this item, first ask yourself whether any barriers are present that the child must overcome to continue playing. Then, observe the parent's/caregiver's actions: Do they assist the child, give scaffolding, or use cues to help the child overcome barriers or obstacles? Barriers may be physical, cognitive, or emotional.	**0 (low)**—Parent/caregiver does not seem aware of the various obstacles or barriers that their child encounters. Or, it seems as though they are interested only in the child's physical safety, which, by itself, creates a barrier to the play. **1 (mild)**—Parent/caregiver focuses on only some of the various obstacles or barriers that their child encounters during play. If the parent/caregiver decides to react, it seems late or not adequate or sensitive to the child's needs or preferences. **2 (moderate)**—Parent/caregiver intermittently fails to respond; responds to a clear situation; or their response seems to be a little too hasty and does not give the child a chance to try for themself. A score that falls in the moderate category lacks the sensitive attunement required to support the child to persist playing. **3 (high)**—Parent/caregiver supports their child in overcoming obstacles and assists only if there is a clear indication that the child may need help. When helping their child, the parent/caregiver uses the right amount and type of assistance needed.

(Continued)

TABLE 4.1. Scoring Guidelines *(Cont.)*

Item Description	Rating Scale Description
4. Parent/caregiver demonstrates *positive affect* during play. Your overall impression of the degree to which the parent's/caregiver's affect is positive. This can range from a parent or caregiver who seems apathetic or unhappy to a parent/caregiver who shows obvious signs of being satisfied, happy, and joyful. Please note that not all kinds of play result in exuberance. An adult engaged with a child in table-top or similar activities not expected to engender exuberance is expected to score a 2.	**0 (low)**—Apathetic or disinterested, may show negative affect (sadness, anger). **1 (low)**—Fairly neutral, or parent's/caregiver's behavior does not completely match with their emotional tone. **2 (moderate)**—Seems to be enjoying self and is relaxed or comfortable with the situation and content and pleased with the child's play. **3 (high)**—Exuberant; giggles, laughs, may sing.
5. Parent/caregiver *supports* the child in *decision making.* Parent/caregiver actively allows the child to decide what to do, offers suggestions, or both. At times, the parent/caregiver may share decision making with the child, *as the situation requires*. The child's actions do not have to be purposeful (e.g., a child can wander while deciding what to do next), but there is a clear sense that they *can* choose and decide by themself or together with the parent/caregiver.	**0 (low)**—Parent/caregiver does not promote the child's ability to decide what to do; their behavior may seem intrusive and interferes with the child's desire to decide what to do. Parent takes over the decision making. **1 (mild)**—Parent/caregiver seems insensitive to the child's wishes or needs to choose for themself. Parent/caregiver does not take over but also does not actively support child's decision-making ability. **2 (moderate)**—Parent/caregiver is clearly trying to support the child's need to decide what to do, promote shared decision making, or both. However, sometimes they may fail in doing so, and their actions may seem a little too controlling or a little unengaged for the situation (a slight lack of attunement). **3 (high)**—There is a clear feeling that the parent/caregiver is interested in promoting their child's ability to initiate, elaborate, and choose play themes, materials, and activities. Parent's/caregiver's intentions and actions indicate that they are interested in making a shared decision on their mutual play when it is indicated.
6. Parent/caregiver provides *a sense of safety* during play, so the child will feel sufficiently safe (emotionally and physically) to keep playing (e.g., selecting toys, coming up with ideas, making modifications, feeling safe to make choices or move around). The parent/caregiver does not interfere unless the child shows clear signs of being distressed, in need of help, or in imminent danger.	**0 (low)**—Parent/caregiver seems unaware of the child's sense of safety or prohibits activities because the parent feels they are too risky. **1 (mild)**—Parent/caregiver is aware of the need to support the child's sense of safety. However, they may have a delayed response or respond in an inappropriate manner. **2 (moderate)**—Parent/caregiver identifies, most of the time, any sense of insecurity in the play session. The parent/caregiver then offers the child assistance to maintain the child's sense of safety, alters the environment, or both. **3 (high)**—Parent/caregiver can easily sense situations in which the child might feel insecure or unsafe. It seems as though the parent/caregiver is attuned to the child's sense of safety. When required, they can respond in a sensitive and caring way that suits the situation and ameliorates the child's sense of insecurity.

(Continued)

TABLE 4.1. Scoring Guidelines *(Cont.)*

Item Description	Rating Scale Description
7. Parent/caregiver *supports* the child's *modifications* or their need to *modify* the activity to maintain the challenge or make it more fun. The activity evolves in some way. However, modifications can be small or subtle. Children enjoy an increase in the challenge or complexity of the activity; however, some children must make a task easier to succeed at it. Your impression should be based on the parent's/caregiver's ability to support the child's need in amount and type of modifications to keep them interested.	**0 (low)**—Parent/caregiver does not allow the child to modify or fails to modify as needed to make the activity more fun for the child. **1 (mild)**—Parent/caregiver does not detect the right time for modifications to suit the child's needs and preferences or discourages the child from making modifications. Often, this results in the child becoming disinterested or frustrated. **2 (moderate)**—Parent/caregiver identifies opportunities for modifications or supports the child's modifications; however, these do not come easily or do not always match the child's preferences or needs. **3 (high)**—Parent/caregiver spontaneously and effortlessly supports modifications the child makes or helps them with modifying activities, if needed. The modifications seem effortless.
8. Parent/caregiver *supports the child in interacting with objects* during play. This can refer to when the parent/caregiver is introducing objects to the child (e.g., when the child is not able to reach for them or needs help to use the object well). The parent/caregiver should not present too many options (toys or ideas on how to use them) at once or impose their ideas for using objects "properly" on the child.	**0 (low)**—Parent/caregiver does not support the child's need to interact with objects or interferes when the child is engaged in any interaction with objects. **1 (mild)**—Parent/caregiver does not detect the right time to support the child while interacting with objects. **2 (moderate)**—Parent/caregiver is aware of the need to support the child's interaction with objects during play. However, sometimes their actions do not match the child's interests or are not sufficiently attuned to or interfere with the play. **3 (high)**—Parent/caregiver continuously supports interaction with objects as needed to match the child's preferences and promote the activity.
9. Parent/caregiver *supports* the child's *transition* from one activity to the other when the first no longer evolves or suits the child's preferences or needs or supports the child to remain with an activity that is meeting the child's needs. Your overall impression of the ease with which the parent/caregiver supports the child's transition from one activity to the other when one has ended or is not evolving and another is available. Assess the parent's/caregiver's ability to detect the need for a transition according to the child's needs and preferences but to not transition too quickly.	**0 (low)**—Parent/caregiver does not support the child's needs to transition between activities or forces transition too quickly. **1 (mild)**—Parent/caregiver redirects the child in a manner that does not suit the child's needs and interferes with the flow of play. **2 (moderate)**—Parent/caregiver supports child's transitions from one activity to the other. Parent/caregiver identifies the right moments to redirect the child to a new activity if needed or does not redirect if the child remains engaged. Parent/caregiver acts with relative ease or only slight reluctance, but the transition is not seamless or occurs a little too quickly. **3 (high)**—Parent/caregiver supports child's transitions or can adapt to the situation or activity to meet the child's needs. In a situation in which a transition is needed, but the child is having difficulty initiating one, parent/caregiver easily redirects or offers different activities. Transitions are seamless or, when transitions are not needed, parent/caregiver promotes continued engagement.

(Continued)

TABLE 4.1. Scoring Guidelines *(Cont.)*

Item Description	Rating Scale Description
10. Parent/caregiver *supports* the child's *negotiations* to have their desires met in a suitable, respectful, and age-appropriate manner. Your overall impression of the ease and finesse with which the parent/caregiver verbally or nonverbally supports the child's negotiation bids. May be particularly evident between play frames, when there is a need to negotiate actions or scenarios, or when something happens that the child is unhappy about. This item includes parent/caregiver support of the child in giving readily understandable cues (facial, verbal, body). *Note.* Parent/caregiver may do so by mimicking, acknowledging, or validating the child's facial expressions, such as smiling, frowning ("I see you are smiling," "You are happy," "You throw the ball away; you do not want to play with it anymore," "I see you are tired; you are rubbing your eyes," "You look disappointed; do you want to try another toy or game?").	**0 (low)**—Parent/caregiver imposes their own will or stops the child from negotiating. **1 (mild)**—Parent/caregiver supports the child's negotiations but seems reluctant to do so. **2 (moderate)**—Parent/caregiver uses moderately skilled strategies (e.g., simple verbal statements, simple gestures) to support the child's negotiation, but efforts seem a little awkward. **3 (high)**—Parent/caregiver supports child's negotiation in a suitable, respectful, and age-appropriate manner.
11. Parent/caregiver *supports* the child's needs in *social play*. Ranges from the parent/caregiver who does not recognize the child's need for interaction to a parent/caregiver who is deeply involved in social play. Parent/caregiver and child are engaged in a *reciprocal exchange* during play. Each one lets their partner finish their action and responds as well. There is a sense of synchronicity. Includes the ease with which the parent/caregiver *initiates* a new play activity with the child and *shares* equipment or ideas with the child during play.	**0 (low)**—Parent/caregiver does not support social play. Parent/caregiver is more of an observer than a playmate or plays in a parallel fashion. There is no awareness of the need for reciprocity. Parent/caregiver seems unaware that they possess something that the child would like to use. **1 (mild)**—Parent/caregiver often fails to support the child's initiations or indications for social play. That may include the following: Parent/caregiver interacts in a neutral way, sometimes interacts in discouraging ways, or fails to interact. Parent/caregiver shares inconsistently or shares a little too readily. There is mild evidence of reciprocity. **2 (moderate)**—Parent/caregiver is aware of the child's need to play interactively. However, sometimes they fail or misinterpret the child's initiations, or their responses may seem a little awkward. May include the following behaviors: Parent/caregiver initiates play, but cues are not clear enough for the child to pick up; parent/caregiver shares consistently but seems reluctant or awkward; and the level of reciprocity is moderate in terms of content. If the adult does not consistently support social play, the level of the child's enjoyment or engagement is only fair. **3 (high)**—The play activity would change dramatically if the parent/caregiver being observed were not present. May include the following: Parent/caregiver initiates play effortlessly (e.g., begins an activity that the child follows readily) or they readily follow child's lead; the parent's/caregiver's actions are attuned with the child's needs and preferences; parent/caregiver easily and consistently shares objects, equipment, or ideas with the child; or the interaction seems highly reciprocal. There are clear indications of give-and-take moments throughout the session. When reciprocity is effective and consistent, both the parent/caregiver and the child are apt to clearly enjoy each other's company.

(Continued)

TABLE 4.1. Scoring Guidelines *(Cont.)*

Item Description	Rating Scale Description
12. Parent/caregiver *supports* the child's engagement in playful *mischief, clowning,* or *joking,* or the parent/caregiver incorporates playful *mischief, clowning,* or *joking* during the play. In situations in which the parent/caregiver incorporates mischief or attempts to be playful (act silly), score your overall impression of how much it supports the child's play. Remember, the intent of mischief is to create fun rather than to physically or emotionally hurt. Parent/caregiver supports the child and uses humor during mutual play, such as exaggerated, swaggering behavior or telling jokes or funny stories. Both joking and clowning are especially, but not necessarily only, for the purpose of engaging the child in play or distracting them if needed. Clowning, especially, can be a part of pretend play. *Note.* It is important to note that not all kinds of play call for mischief, teasing, or joking. In those cases, score this item N/A.	**0 (low)**—Parent's/caregiver's attempts at mischief seem more to annoy or divert the child's attention to the parent/caregiver than to increase everyone's fun in the context of the play activity, or parent/caregiver does not support the child's engagement in playful mischief even when child's attempts at mischief seem warranted and fun. **1 (mild)**—Parent/caregiver picks up some of the child's playful and mischievous behaviors but responds in a less-than-attuned manner. Parent/caregiver carries out mischief, but it lacks a sensitive match with the child's needs. **2 (moderate)**—Parent/caregiver picks up the child's playful, mischievous behaviors and joins in but may seem a little awkward or reluctant to join in. **3 (high)**—Parent/caregiver carries out sophisticated mischief, turns mischief into play, and gets the child to laugh; mischief defuses a potentially difficult situation and creates fun. It is attuned to the child's and the dyad's needs. Or the parent/caregiver is supportive of the child's playful and mischievous behaviors.
13. Parent/caregiver *supports* the child's *pretending* (to be someone else; to do something else; that an object is something else; that something else is happening). Parent/caregiver may enter into the pretend play as well. Your overall impression is of the degree to which the adult's actions support the child's pretend behavior. *Note.* It is important to note that not all kinds of play call for pretending, and some very young children would not be expected to engage in pretend play yet, developmentally. In those cases, score this item N/A.	**0 (low)**—Parent/caregiver does not support the child's engagement in pretend play; the parent/caregiver may suggest a different activity. **1 (mild)**—Parent's/caregiver's initiations in pretend play are not at all convincing. **2 (moderate)**—Parent/caregiver acts in a way that says they are aware of the advantages that pretend play holds for the child and their mutual play. Parent's/caregiver's pretend actions are mildly to moderately convincing or a little awkward. **3 (high)**—Parent's/caregiver's actions are highly convincing. It seems as though the parent/caregiver is attuned to the child's needs and thus uses pretend play to engage the child, create more fun, and/or defuse stressful moments. Parent/caregiver seamlessly supports the child's pretending in play.

(Continued)

TABLE 4.1. Scoring Guidelines *(Cont.)*

Item Description	Rating Scale Description
14. Parent/caregiver *supports* or encourages the child to *incorporate* objects or other people into play in *unconventional or variable* ways. Parent/caregiver supports or encourages the child to look for possibilities within a toy, object, or another person. For example, they may use objects commonly thought of as toys in ways other than those the manufacturer clearly intended or cast people in nonhuman roles, incorporate objects not classically thought of as toys into the play (e.g., bugs, table legs), or use one toy or object in a few different ways. Your overall impression of the *ease* with which the parent/caregiver incorporates objects or other people in variable or creative ways. *Note.* It is important to note that, as with pretend play, not all kinds of play call for using objects or people in unconventional play. In those cases, score this item NA.	**0 (low)**—Parent/caregiver does not support or discourages the child from incorporating objects or other people into play in unconventional or variable ways. **1 (mild)**—Parent/caregiver supports child's use of objects in slightly different ways. Parent/caregiver does not encourage the child to look for other possibilities within an object, other than what the child produced, or they do so in an inappropriate manner that does not meet the child's capabilities. **2 (moderate)**—Parent/caregiver supports the child's usage of objects and/or other people in moderately unconventional or creative ways or parent/caregiver contributes to other options for the child to pick up. **3 (high)**—Parent/caregiver seems aware of the gains and developmental advantages of using objects, toys, or people in an unconventional way. Thus, they easily support and incorporate objects in creative ways that are attuned with the child's needs, preferences, and capabilities.
15. Parent/caregiver adheres to *consistent, reasonable, and clear boundaries or rules.* Rules do not change unexpectedly. *Note.* When examiners notice that a child is disinterested or fatigued, it *may be* that the rules are not reasonable, and the parent/caregiver continues to elicit a response from them. This may be evident in situations in which the parent/caregiver reinforces rules or boundaries. Sometimes it may stem from a parent's/caregiver's inability to capture the child's motivation, and instead they reinforce rules.	**0 (low)**—Parent's/caregiver's boundaries or rules seem unreasonable or harsh at times, or they keep changing them in an unexpected manner. While the child is engaged in something, the parent/caregiver will not allow the play to continue although there are no apparent safety issues. For example, parent/caregiver insists that the child play with a toy only in the way the manufacturer intended. **1 (low/mild)**—Parent/caregiver does not provide consistent, clear, or reasonable boundaries or rules to the child. Parent/caregiver exhibits overriding behavior without being aware of it. **2 (moderate)**—Parent/caregiver sets reasonable and consistent boundaries or rules that seem appropriate ("Let's put this piece here, then that one"; the parent/caregiver does not allow the child to throw toys on the floor when the child is frustrated). Parent/caregiver rarely exhibits overriding behavior; if such behavior is present, it is only for a moment. **3 (high)**—Parent/caregiver sets appropriate limits to the child's behavior. The limit setting seems reasonable, clear, and consistent. Parent/caregiver redirects the child when it is beneficial to the child's play. Parent/caregiver does not display controlling behavior.

(Continued)

TABLE 4.1. Scoring Guidelines *(Cont.)*

Item Description	Rating Scale Description
16. Parent/caregiver *verbally praises* the child for a desired and appropriate behavior during play interactions. *Note.* Praise is often most appropriate in situations in which a parent/caregiver is teaching a child to do something in the context of the play or when the adult is surprised by a child's action or accomplishment. If praise does not seem appropriate for the play situation, then score NA.	**0 (low)**—Parent/caregiver does not praise the child or seems unaware of the need for and benefits of praising the child's behavior or accomplishments. **1 (mild)**—Parent/caregiver uses praise generally ("good job"), or praise seems to disrupt the flow of the play. **2 (moderate)**—Parent/caregiver praises the child's behavior specifically ("You did a great job; you built such a nice tower") or primarily provides general praise ("Good boy," "Good girl"). **3 (high)**—Parent/caregiver verbally and specifically praises the child for a desired and appropriate behavior during play interactions (e.g., parent/caregiver praises the child when they show effort in accomplishing a task).

TABLE 4.2. Scoring Form

Dyad (#): **Age:** **Rater:** **In** **Out** **Video** **Live** **(Circle)**		**Scale** **NA = not applicable** **0 = low** **1 = mild** **2 = moderate** **3 = high**
Items	**Score**	**Comments**
1. Parent/caregiver is *actively supporting* the child's engagement in free play.		
2. Parent/caregiver supports the child's engagement in the activity *for the process* rather than primarily for the end product (building, assembling, and "getting the job done").		
3. Parent/caregiver *helps* the child *overcome barriers or obstacles* to persist with the activity.		
4. Parent/caregiver demonstrates *positive affect* during play.		
5. Parent/caregiver *supports* the child in *decision making*.		
6. Parent/caregiver provides *a sense of safety* during play, so the child will feel sufficiently safe (emotionally and physically) to keep playing (e.g., selecting toys, coming up with ideas, making modifications, feeling safe to make choices or move around).		
7. Parent/caregiver *supports* the child's *modifications* or their need to *modify* the activity to maintain the challenge or make it more fun.		
8. Parent/caregiver *supports the child in interacting with objects* during play.		
9. Parent/caregiver *supports* the child's *transition* from one activity to the other when the first no longer evolves or suits the child's preferences or needs or supports the child to remain with an activity that is meeting the child's needs.		

(Continued)

TABLE 4.2. Scoring Form *(Cont.)*

Items	Score	Comments
10. Parent/caregiver *supports* the child's *negotiations* to have their desires met in a suitable, respectful, and age-appropriate manner.		
11. Parent/caregiver *supports* the child's need in *social play*.		
12. Parent/caregiver *supports* the child's engagement in playful *mischief, clowning*, or *joking*, or the parent/caregiver incorporates *mischief, clowning, or joking* during play.		
13. Parent/caregiver *supports* the child's *pretending* (to be someone else; to do something else; that an object is something else; that something else is happening). Parent/caregiver may enter into the pretend play as well.		
14. Parent/caregiver *supports* or encourages the child to *incorporate* objects or other people into play in *unconventional or variable* ways.		
15. Parent/caregiver adheres to *consistent, reasonable, and clear boundaries or rules*. Rules do not change unexpectedly.		
16. Parent/caregiver *verbally praises* the child for a desired and appropriate behavior during play interactions.		
Average score	**Sum of column scores/16 or number of items scored, excluding items scored NA**	

Interpretation of Scores

After scoring the PC-SCP, the examiner can interpret the findings in two ways.

1. First, examine the scoring profile (i.e., pattern of scores), and consider the caregiving role and behaviors the adult is exhibiting in the transaction.
2. Second, use the key form, shown in Figure 4.1, to get a sense of how this dyad's scores compare with those of others who have taken the PC-SCP. (The key form is also available in Appendix B.)

SCORING PROFILE

If the majority of scores are 0 or 1, consider assessing the child's playfulness in the same environment, and perhaps also in a different one, using the Test of Playfulness (ToP; see Skard & Bundy, 2008) to better understand the child's playfulness and contributions to the joint play. If the ToP reveals deficits in one or more elements of playfulness, then the practitioner should consider the need for direct services to the child. However, because playfulness is so environmentally dependent, we believe that dyadic sessions to assist the parent or caregiver and child to engage in joint play are the preferred intervention. If the ToP reveals that the child does not exhibit challenges in their playfulness behavior in other circumstances, then the focus of the intervention would be on assisting the parent or caregiver to improve their level of support, incorporating consultation. Again, engaging in dyadic sessions (perhaps videotaped) followed by consultation is the preferred intervention.

A scoring profile with most scores being 2 or 3 indicates that the parent or caregiver demonstrates behavior supportive of the child's play and playfulness. In that case, there is no indication of a need to provide services. However, if the parent or caregiver expresses a need to learn more about how to engage the child in different forms of play, then the practitioner can provide consultation directed to the dyad or the parent's or caregiver's needs. Further examples of PC–SCP profiles and guidance on play-based intervention are provided in Chapter 5.

CAREGIVING BEHAVIORS AND ROLES

Sethi's (2020) conceptualization of caregiving roles and behaviors, described briefly in Chapter 2, can assist in understanding parents' or caregivers' supportiveness and needs. Here we suggest three roles derived from Sethi's work to understand joint play. The examiner can review the PC–SCP scoring profile and identify whether the parent or caregiver experienced particular challenges in one or more of the following:

- *Caregiver and protector:* keeping the child safe and feeling secure by providing clear and consistent boundaries and a safe play environment (see Items 1, 2, 5, 6, and 15).
- *Nurturer:* showing affection and expressing love and care toward the child as well as constructive feedback or praise (see Items 4 and 16, as well as the overall impression of this joint play experience).
- *Educator and learner:* focusing on (positive) change in the child's behavior by assisting the child to behave differently or learn a new skill (i.e., manipulating toys or ideas, communicating needs, transitioning between play activities; see Items 3, 7, 8, 9, 10, 11, 12, 13, and 14) and learning from the child and supporting them as they engage in joint play, using strategies such as self-correction, mental talk ("I see you want to continue playing; that's okay, we can finish the puzzle later"); see overall scoring within the range of 2 to 3 points.

USING THE KEY FORM

The key form, shown in Figure 4.1, allows examiners to compare a dyad's score with those of others who have taken the PC–SCP. To use the key form, the examiner circles the score awarded for each item and then draws a median line through the scores so that half the scores are above the line and half are below. Next, the examiner extends the line to the right side of the key form. This line will pass through the overall PC–SCP raw score, the measure score, and the standard error calculated in the Rasch analysis to the asterisks representing scores of the data sample. The examiner can then see how the dyad's scores compare with those of the data sample.

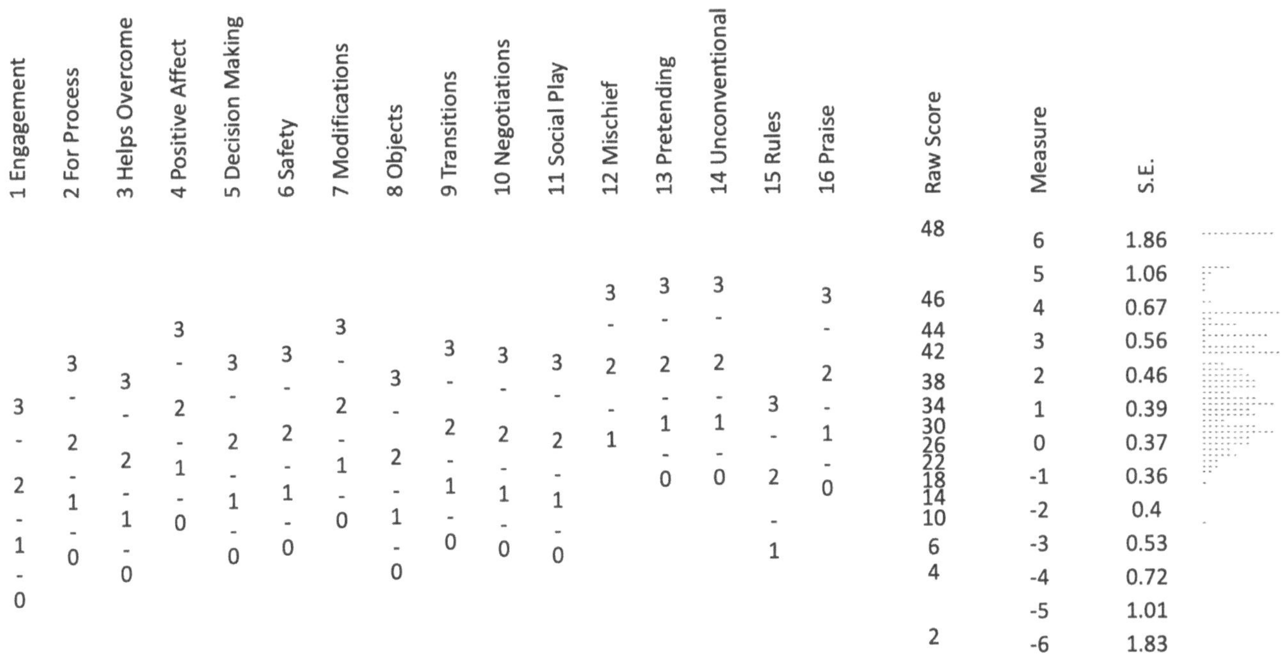

Figure 4.1 Key form.

5

Clinical Application and Case Examples

The following five case examples illustrate PC–SCP scoring based on observing joint play interactions between a parent and a child in their home. Among the five cases, there are three mother–child dyads and two father–child dyads. The children's ages range from 2 to 9 years. Each case includes brief background information, an observation transcript, and a PC–SCP scoring form with examples from the transcript to support the scoring. Each case concludes with a summary of caregiver and protector, nurturer, and educator and learner behaviors and directions for intervention.

Karla and Martin

Karla is age 34 years and a single mother. She works full time as a store manager. Her son, **Martin,** is age 2 years. He attends daycare when Karla is at work. Martin achieved all developmental milestones on time. However, Karla asked for an evaluation by an occupational therapist because she was worried about his attention span and noncompliant behavior. Martin's preferred language is English.

JOINT PLAY OBSERVATION

Karla and Martin were observed playing at Martin's grandmother's house, where they both live. They played in a space where they usually play. The session began with Martin drawing an image on the table while standing and Karla asking, "What are you doing? Can I draw too?" Martin responded, "Yes," and both began drawing together. A little while later, Karla sorted cards while Martin continued drawing (observer's note: The mother does not seem to be paying attention to the child). Karla said to Martin, "What else you wanna do?" Martin did not respond but continued drawing, dropping a crayon on the floor. Karla: "Look, it's by my foot." Martin got down on the floor, picked it up, and continued to draw. When Martin sneezed, Karla said, "God bless you! Say 'thank you!'" Martin still did not respond and continued to draw. Karla then looked up from sorting the cards, made a cringing facial expression, and said to Martin, "You stink" (observer's note: She tried to play with him but drifted away because he had an accident). Karla looked at the camera and covered her mouth. She then looked at Martin and said, "Look at the ball. Pick it up and put it into the basket!" When Martin complied, Karla said, "Good job." She gave Martin a high five and called him a "superstar." After putting the ball into the basket, Martin resumed drawing, while Karla picked up the cards and asked if he wanted to learn some Spanish. She began naming the numbers out loud in English and Spanish, but Martin did not repeat them. Karla continued naming the numbers, but Martin still did not respond. Martin then turned around and hit the card out of Karla's hand. She responded by saying, "Don't hit it off my hand!" Martin went back to drawing. Karla picked up the blue crayon and told him to draw the image blue. He took the crayon from her and colored with it.

Martin began drawing with a yellow crayon while Karla sat on the couch. She picked up a truck (observer's note: in an effort to get Martin's attention). Martin turned around and looked at the truck. Karla began playing with the truck on the table and on the floor. Martin then went to the truck and kicked it. Karla responded, "Don't kick it. Not nice." Karla then got another car and played with it (observer's note: Martin ignored it) while Martin returned to drawing. Karla asked, "Can I draw with you?" and then, "Why do you keep dropping everything to the floor? Pick it up. The cap is over here." Martin picked up all the items from the floor and then grabbed the yellow crayon and continued to draw. Karla lay on the couch for about a minute and then sat up (observer's note: she seemed to be bored and not interested in playing). Karla then grabbed some of the blocks and placed them on the table next to Martin (observer's note: Karla seemed interested, but Martin did not want to play with her. It seemed like he would rather continue coloring). Martin grabbed the blocks, put them back, and continued coloring. Karla touched Martin's hair and asked, "Can I color?" She tried to grab the crayon from his hand, and Martin screamed, "No!" Karla responded, "That's not nice!" and Martin continued to draw on his own. Scoring for Karla and Martin is shown in Table 5.1.

TABLE 5.1. Karla and Martin PC–SCP Scoring

Dyad (#): Karla and Martin	**Scale**
Age:	**NA = not applicable** **0 = low** **1 = mild**
Rater:	**2 = moderate** **3 = high**
In **Out** **Video** **Live** **(Circle)**	

Items	**Score**	**Comments**
1. Parent/caregiver is *actively supporting* the child's engagement in free play.	1	Karla does not seem to be attuned to Martin's needs. There are times when she is engaged, and at other times she redirects his attention to activities she wants him to do. "What are you doing? Can I draw too?" Both the child and the mother begin drawing together. Karla is then seen sorting cards while Martin continues drawing. Karla tries to grab the crayon from his hand, and Martin screams, "No!"
2. Parent/caregiver supports the child's engagement in the activity *for the process* rather than primarily for the end product (building, assembling, and "getting the job done").	1	Karla encourages task-oriented behaviors. She begins to name the numbers out loud in both languages, but he does not repeat the numbers. Karla continues to name the numbers out loud, but Martin still does not respond.
3. Parent/caregiver *helps* the child *overcome barriers or obstacles* to persist with the activity.	1	Karla assists Martin to get toys or objects that are out of reach. "While Martin is drawing, he drops the crayon on the floor and Karla says, "Look, it's by my foot."
4. Parent/caregiver demonstrates *positive affect* during play.	0	Negative affect or seems bored throughout.
5. Parent/caregiver *supports* the child in *decision making*.	2	Asks Martin questions to verify his preferences. Sometimes it is a distraction; at other times, it supports Martin's decision-making ability.
6. Parent/caregiver *provides a sense of safety* during play, so the child will feel sufficiently safe (emotionally and physically) to keep playing (e.g., selecting toys, coming up with ideas, making modifications, feeling safe to make choices or move around).	1	Overall, she is in close proximity to child but ignoring his cues regarding what he wants to do and seems to interfere with his feelings of safety to continue playing.

(Continued)

TABLE 5.1. PC–SCP Scoring for Karla and Martin *(Cont.)*

Items	Score	Comments
7. Parent/caregiver *supports* child's *modifications* or their need to *modify* the activity to maintain the challenge or make it more fun.	1	Martin does not try to modify it, and Karla's changing activities likely interfere with that.
8. Parent/caregiver *supports the child in interacting with objects* during play.	2	Karla supports Martin by trying to direct him toward playing with the ball: "Look at the ball. Pick it up and put it into the basket!" Martin does it. But other times she tries to change the activity when he seems to want to continue.
9. Parent/caregiver *supports* the child's *transition* from one activity to the other when the first no longer evolves or suits the child's preferences or needs or supports the child to remain with an activity that is meeting the child's needs.	1	Asks questions about what Martin is playing with or suggests a change that does not match the child's interests or actions.
10. Parent/caregiver *supports* the child's *negotiations* to have their desires met in a suitable, respectful, and age-appropriate manner.	2	Karla is interested in what Martin is doing or if he wants to play with something else but seems to ignore his cues that he wants to keep drawing.
11. Parent/caregiver *supports* the child's needs in *social play*.	2	Karla tries to engage Martin in social play: "Can I draw with you?" (Asked couple of times throughout the observation). She begins to name the numbers out loud in both languages, but he does not join in.
12. Parent/caregiver *supports* the child's engagement in playful *mischief, clowning,* or *joking,* or the parent/caregiver incorporates *mischief, clowning, or joking* during play.	NA	No playful mischief behavior was observed.
13. Parent/caregiver *supports* the child's *pretending* (to be someone else; to do something else; that an object is something else; that something else is happening). Parent/caregiver may enter into the pretend play as well.	NA	No pretend play was observed, but Martin is only 2, and the activities in which they are engaging do not really support pretend play.
14. Parent/caregiver *supports* or encourages the child to *incorporate* objects or other people into play in *unconventional or variable* ways.	NA	The activities in which they are engaging do not really support unconventional play.
15. Parent/caregiver adheres to *consistent, reasonable, and clear boundaries or rules.* Rules do not change unexpectedly.	2	Keeps clear boundaries.
16. Parent/caregiver *verbally praises* the child for a desired and appropriate behavior during play interactions.	1	Karla gives the child a high five and calls him a "superstar."
Average score	**Sum of column scores/16 or number of items scored, excluding items scored NA**	**17/13 = 1.3**

SCORING REASONING

- *Caregiver and protector:* task-oriented behaviors geared toward educating Martin and only partially addressing his preferences or needs (see Items 1, 2, and 5). Karla kept in close physical proximity, which allowed her to ensure Martin's safety. She provided clear and direct guidance; however, there was little evidence of her attending to Martin's play cues (see Items 6 and 15).
- *Nurturer:* little affection or nurturing expressed toward the child; however, Karla provided some age-appropriate praise (see Items 4 and 16).
- *Educator and learner:* Karla provided Martin with support during the joint play interaction aimed at either teaching him what she thought was important or assisting him in completing a task. Her educational efforts were not child centered or geared toward Martin's needs or toward promoting play (see Items 3, 7, 8, 9, 10, 11, 12, 13, and 14). There was no evidence of self-correction strategies or mental talk (see overall scores within the range of 2–3 points).

SUGGESTIONS FOR INTERVENTION

- Help Karla to understand the reasons for Martin's apparent noncompliance. Some are age related; some may stem from their interactions.
- Discuss the importance of child-directed play and ways for Karla to continue educating her son while adjusting the activities to fit his needs and interests. Discuss the differences between, and advantages of, both child-directed and parent-directed play.
- Help Karla recognize and respond to Martin's cues.
- Discuss ways to create a balance between child-directed and parent-directed play so they can have fun and enjoy joint play.
- Model ways of communication in which guidance and help are less directive to allow Martin to explore new ideas and figure out problems during the play.

Melissa and Charlie

Melissa is age 41 years and married with four children. She works full-time as a nurse. **Charlie,** age 4 years, 2 months, is Melissa's youngest child. He achieved all developmental milestones on time. Melissa has sought an occupational therapy evaluation for Charlie because he mostly plays by himself and has a hard time playing with his older siblings, who like to play board games. She was concerned Charlie might have learning difficulties. Charlie attends preschool. His preferred language is English.

JOINT PLAY OBSERVATION

Melissa and Charlie were observed playing at home in a space where they usually play. The session began with Melissa and Charlie playing a board game at the table. Charlie rolled the dice, and Melissa said, "Five, two, oh my god, you got five. So, you come out." They both look at each other, and Melissa encouraged Charlie to move his pawn. Melissa then said, "And then you do two—one and two." Charlie took his pawn out and started moving it around the board. Melissa told him to go back to where he started and pointed to where he needed to move his pawn. Once he corrected it, she said, "Yes, you stay there. Now it is my turn." She picked up the dice. Charlie looked at his mother, rubbed his hands together (observer's note: as if he has a plan), and laughed. Melissa said, "You're out first. That's not fair!" Melissa then rolled the dice. She put her hands up, saying, "I'm out too. Five, one, two, three." She moved her pawn, and Charlie giggled. Melissa then looked up at the camera and smiled.

Melissa handed the dice to Charlie, and he rolled. She asked, "Okay, how much is that?" Charlie leaned over the board and said, "Hmm." Pointing to the dice, Melissa reiterated, "How much is this? This plus this is how much?" Charlie responded, "Hmm . . . three?" Melissa: "Yes, so you go. And this one?" Charlie answered, "Two." Melissa then specified, "So you're gonna do three first." She picked up his pawn. As he moved it, she counted for him. Then she said, "You know how to count. One. . . ." Charlie began counting with her. She took the pawn from him, saying, "No, one, two. . . ." The child continued, "Two, three, four, five" as Melissa moved his pawn. She confirmed, saying, "Yes." Melissa then said, "Okay, you are getting there. Every box is one, Charlie." She pointed to a box, then picked up her finger and showed him the number one. She then accidentally dropped the dice and bent down to pick it up. Charlie looked under the table to see what she was doing. He went under the table, picked up the dice, and handed it to his mother. Melissa rolled, repeating, "So every box is one." Charlie looked at the camera and smiled.

Melissa proceeded, "Okay, my turn." She rolled and then said, "Okay. I'm coming out." She moved her pawn, saying, "Five. You see?" She pointed to the dice, moved the pawn five spots and said "One, two." Charlie laughed. Melissa handed the dice to Charlie, saying with a smile, "Now your turn. I gotta move before you kill me." Melissa pointed to the dice after Charlie rolled and asked him, "You have how much?" Charlie pointed to the dice, saying, "Two and two." Melissa responded, "Okay, so you go." Charlie moved his pawn two spots. Melissa questioned, "Mm, and what else?" Charlie looked at Melissa and she asked, "How many times?" Charlie moved the pawn one spot forward. Melissa questioned, "Mm . . .?" and Charlie moved the pawn another spot forward. Melissa responded cheerfully, "Yes. Very good."

Melissa picked up the dice and explained, "Now, this is a double. When you have a double, you gotta play again." He responded (observer's note: understandingly), "Again. Oooohhh." Melissa confirmed, "Yes, you gotta roll the dice . . . roll it . . . Oh my god." She fumbled with the dice and continued, "You gotta do it again. Here." She handed Charlie the dice, and he rolled. Melissa asked, "Okay, so what you got?" She pointed to the dice. Charlie responded, "Double?" Melissa explained, "No, it's not a double. What is this?" She moved the dice toward him. He leaned over the table and hesitated, "Ummmm." Melissa pointed to the dice asking, "Can you come out with this?" Charlie questioned, "Five?" She responded, "Yes." Charlie then added, "And six." Melissa: (observer's note: cheered), "Yessss, give me a high five. Good! That's my son!" They high fived each other, and then Charlie smiled.

Melissa then asked, "So, how you come out? What are you gonna use to come out?" Charlie questioned, "Ummmmm?" and she responded, "Remember, how you come out?" She pointed to the dice, asking, "What do you need to come out?" Charlie, still thinking, repeated "Ummmm," and Melissa explained, "Five, right?" She grabbed his pawn and moved it out for him. She then pointed to the other dice and said, "And how you gonna get six? Move this one and then move this one. Whatever you want." She pointed to his pawn and then rolled the dice. Charlie looked at his mother (observer's note: for confirmation) as he moved his pieces forward. She counted with him, "One, two, three . . . see it? Four. . . ." He moved the pawn as she counted. He continued moving his pawn, and Melissa said, "Yes (observer's note: she confirms).

Melissa rolled the dice. Charlie rubbed his hands together (observer's note: mischievously) and laughed. Melissa: "Okay, five, two. So, Mommy is gonna come out," and they both laughed again. She moved a pawn out. She used her other pawn to count, "One, two." Melissa handed Charlie the dice: "Here you go." He rolled, and she said, "Four, two. Oooo." Pointing to his two pawns, Melissa asked, "So how much you gonna get? What you gonna do? This one or this one?" When Charlie responded, "Mmmmhmmmm," Melissa said, "You can use whatever you want. So, count." Charlie moved his pawn. Melissa said (observer's note: explains): "You gotta go this way, not backwards." She pointed in the correct direction. Charlie moved his pawn as he counted, "1, 2, 3, 4, 5, 6." Melissa (observer's note: confirmed): "Yes. You know your numbers. I am so proud." She looked at him and smiled. He smiled back, then laughed. He rubs his hands together as Melissa rolled. She says "Ooooo! Double two-oooo-oooo!" She looked at her son and tapped his nose. He laughed. Melissa counted as she moved her pawn. She said "I gotta do it again." Charlie made a funny sound as he waited. They continued the game cheerfully. Scoring for Melissa and Charlie is shown in Table 5.2.

TABLE 5.2. Melissa and Charlie PC–SCP Scoring

Dyad (#): Melissa and Charlie **Age:** **Rater:** **In Out Video Live (Circle)**	**Scale** **NA = not applicable** **0 = low** **1 = mild** **2 = moderate** **3 = high**	
Items	**Score**	**Comments**
1. Parent/caregiver is *actively supporting* the child's engagement in free play.	3	Melissa is actively engaged throughout the entire time they were observed playing.
2. Parent/caregiver supports the child's engagement in the activity *for the process* rather than primarily for the end product (building, assembling, and "getting the job done").	2	Melissa supports Charlie's engagement in the process of playing, but she is also concerned with teaching Charlie how to count and complete the game they started.
3. Parent/caregiver *helps* the child *overcome barriers or obstacles* to persist with the activity.	3	Melissa supports Charlie when he faces challenges. "This plus this is how much?" she repeats while pointing to one dice. Melissa: "Yes, so you go. And this one?"
4. Parent/caregiver demonstrates *positive affect* during play.	2	There were clear signs of positive affect (they were observed to be playing cheerfully and smiling).
5. Parent/caregiver *supports* the child in *decision making*.	2	Melissa is directing Charlie in making decisions using more general guidance and support. She guides him to a solution rather than letting Charlie figure it out himself.
6. Parent/caregiver *provides a sense of safety* during play, so the child will feel sufficiently safe (emotionally and physically) to keep playing (e.g., selecting toys, coming up with ideas, making modifications, feeling safe to make choices or move around).	3	Melissa's words and actions provide a sense of safety for Charlie.
7. Parent/caregiver *supports* child's *modifications* or their needs to *modify* the activity to maintain the challenge or make it more fun.	NA	Because they are playing a game by the rules, modifications would be uncommon.
8. Parent/caregiver *supports the child in interacting with objects* during play.	2	Sometimes Melissa manipulated objects for him, instead of encouraging Charlie to do it himself.
9. Parent/caregiver *supports* the child's *transition* from one activity to the other when the first no longer evolves or suits the child's preferences or needs or supports the child to remain with an activity that is meeting the child's needs.	3	Melissa's words and actions encouraged Charlie to continue with the game; it suited his interests, and he showed progression in skill and enjoyment.
10. Parent/caregiver *supports* the child's *negotiations* to have their desires met in a suitable, respectful, and age-appropriate manner.	2	There are several examples of back-and-forth verbal interaction, although directive in nature.
11. Parent/caregiver *supports* the child's needs in *social play*.	3	The synchrony between Melissa and Charlie is evident throughout the entire observation.

(Continued)

TABLE 5.2. Melissa and Charlie PC–SCP Scoring *(Cont.)*

Items	Score	Comments
12. Parent/caregiver *supports* the child's engagement in playful *mischief, clowning,* or *joking,* or the parent/caregiver incorporates *mischief, clowning,* or *joking* during play.	NA	Not evident. Games with rules when a child is first learning the game rarely yield a lot of opportunity for mischief.
13. Parent/caregiver *supports* the child's *pretending* (to be someone else; to do something else; that an object is something else; that something else is happening). Parent/caregiver may enter into the pretend play as well.	NA	Games with rules when a child is first learning the game rarely yield a lot of opportunity for pretend.
14. Parent/caregiver *supports* or encourages the child to *incorporate* objects or other people into play in *unconventional or variable* ways.	NA	Again, the nature of the play means that there would be little opportunity for unconventional use of objects or people.
15. Parent/caregiver adheres to *consistent, reasonable, and clear boundaries or rules.* Rules do not change unexpectedly.	3	The rules are clear and appropriate.
16. Parent/caregiver *verbally praises* the child for a desired and appropriate behavior during play interaction.	3	The interaction is warm with multiple examples of praise for effort or capability. "You know your numbers. I am so proud." She looks at him and smiles. He smiles back, then laughs.
Average score	**Sum of column scores/16 or number or items scored, excluding items scored NA**	**32/12 = 2.7**

SCORING REASONING

- *Caregiver and protector:* Melissa is attuned to Charlie's needs and provides help during play when needed (see Items 1, 2, and 5). Melissa provides clear and consistent boundaries; together with her positive affect and supportive presence, she creates a safe and secure environment for Charlie to play in (see Items 6 and 15).
- *Nurturer:* Melissa's positive emotions and her sense of pride when Charlie demonstrates ability were well expressed. It is also important to acknowledge his effort in situations in which he struggles or tries to overcome challenges to continue playing (see Items 4 and 16).
- *Educator and learner:* Melissa is attuned to Charlie's needs and capabilities, demonstrating learning capacity, and provides the amount of support that he needs, which seems to make him feel capable and contributes to self-directed behavior (see Items 3, 7, 8, 9, 10, 11, 12, 13, and 14). The only aspect of play she did not support was pretense and creative play. The board game they played does not necessarily lend itself to that sort of play. Charlie is capable of playing this board game but requires support for counting, which Melissa provided. However, his siblings may not be aware of how to provide it. They may also not be interested in having Charlie join them for all games (scores across the PC–SCP are 2 or 3).

SUGGESTIONS FOR INTERVENTION

- Melissa provided support for Charlie's play in a new game with rules.
- Discuss the difference between child-directed and parent-directed play and the benefits of each, including ways to incorporate pretending and mischief into the play.
- Discuss reasons why Charlie may not play games with siblings and how to promote that if it is important to Charlie.

Matt and Sabrina

Matt is age 38 years and divorced. He works full-time as a banker. **Sabrina,** age 2 years, 7 months, is his only child. Sabrina attends daycare because both her parents work full time. Sabrina reached developmental milestones on time. Sabrina's daycare teacher recommended her parents consult with an occupational therapist because, at the daycare, Sabrina transitions between activities rather quickly compared with her peers. The teacher also added that Sabrina prefers to play with her and the teacher aides rather than with her peers. Her preferred language is English.

JOINT PLAY OBSERVATION

Matt and Sabrina were observed playing at the home where Sabrina lives with her mother. They played together in a bright living room well equipped with toys. The TV was on the entire time. Matt sat on the couch throughout the observation while Sabrina moved around the room.

At first, Sabrina knelt in front of the couch, eating pizza. Then Matt asked Sabrina to make coffee, but she pretended to make pizza instead in a toy kitchen on the other side of the room. Matt joined her, and they played this for about 2 minutes. Then Matt suggested they play ball. Sabrina spent most of the time running after the ball (observer's note: she does not catch or throw the ball well). They played ball for about 2 minutes. Sabrina switched to playing with a large white bin; she sat in it, put it on her head, and then stood on it and jumped off. She did this for about 1 minute. Matt told her multiple times to stop; he did not want her to break the bin or get hurt jumping off it (observer's note: It seems like Sabrina does not know what she wants to play). Matt suggested they sing "The Wheels on the Bus" while Sabrina sat on a small toy bus, which they did for almost 2 minutes. Then Matt asked for hugs, and Sabrina complied. Sabrina then started playing with a doll blanket and a doll and pretended to put her to sleep. She did this for about 2 minutes. Then she found a toy doctor kit and pretended to give shots to her doll, Matt, herself, and the observer; then she asked Matt to give her a shot. They engaged in this play for about 2 minutes. Sabrina then picked up the toy stethoscope and used it on Matt, the observer, and the wall for another 2 minutes. After the doctor play, Sabrina picked up her doll, still lying on the floor, and put it on a mattress so the doll would go to sleep. She played with the doll for about 30 seconds. Sabrina then went back to the toy kitchen for less than a minute; she and Matt talked about what she wanted to make for lunch. The observation ended with Sabrina holding a tool from the doctor kit to test knee reflexes. Matt tried to show her how to use the tool, but Sabrina did not want to give it to him. Table 5.3 shows scoring for Matt and Sabrina.

TABLE 5.3. Matt and Sabrina PC–SCP Scoring

Dyad (#): Matt and Sabrina	Scale
Age:	NA = not applicable 0 = low 1 = mild 2 = moderate 3 = high
Rater:	
In Out Video Live (Circle)	

Items	Score	Comments
1. Parent/caregiver is *actively supporting* the child's engagement in free play.	1	Matt does not seem to be fully engaged in any of the play activities, perhaps contributing to Sabrina's quick transitions between activities.
2. Parent/caregiver supports the child's engagement in the activity *for the process* rather than primarily for the end product (building, assembling, and "getting the job done").	1	Sabrina and Matt are engaged in goal-directed play activities (playing catch, making pizza, and singing a song).
3. Parent/caregiver *helps* the child *overcome barriers or obstacles* to persist with the activity.	1	Sabrina's main barrier is in elaborating play and sustaining her engagement for more than a few minutes. Matt does not seem to be able to identify this obstacle or his potential contributions to it by not getting engaged himself.
4. Parent/caregiver demonstrates *positive affect* during play.	1	Fairly neutral (no laughter, joking around, smiles, etc.); one time Matt asked Sabrina for a hug.
5. Parent/caregiver *supports* the child in *decision making*.	0	Matt does allow Sabrina to make decisions, but he does not help her to follow through and become engaged.
6. Parent/caregiver *provides a sense of safety* during play, so the child will feel sufficiently safe (emotionally and physically) to keep playing (e.g., selecting toys, coming up with ideas, making modifications, feeling safe to make choices or move around).	2	Matt does not want her to break the bin or get hurt by jumping off it and tells her multiple times to stop climbing and jumping on it. Sabrina does feel safe and continues with the activity.
7. Parent/caregiver *supports* the child's *modifications* or their needs to *modify* the activity to maintain the challenge or make it more fun.	1	There is not much support for modifications. Had Matt encouraged modification, each activity might have continued for longer.
8. Parent/caregiver *supports the child in interacting with objects* during play.	1	The support is in simple back-and-forth manipulation of objects. Matt chose not to help Sabrina manipulate the ball more effectively.
9. Parent/caregiver *supports* the child's *transition* from one activity to the other when the first no longer evolves or suits the child's preferences or needs or supports the child to remain with an activity that is meeting the child's needs.	1	Suggests moving between activities too quickly.
10. Parent/caregiver *supports* the child's *negotiations* to have their desires met in a suitable, respectful, and age-appropriate manner.	2	Throughout the observation, Matt was asking and checking what Sabrina wanted to play with.

(Continued)

TABLE 5.3. Matt and Sabrina PC–SCP Scoring *(Cont.)*

Items	Score	Comments
11. Parent/caregiver *supports* the child's needs in *social play*.	1	Brief moments of synchrony tend to stop after a few minutes.
12. Parent/caregiver *supports* the child's engagement in playful *mischief, clowning*, or *joking*, or the parent/caregiver incorporates playful *mischief, clowning, or joking* during play.	1	Although there were opportunities for mischief, Matt did not encourage any. Play with the bin could have been interpreted as mischief if it was genuinely not dangerous, but Matt shut that down.
13. Parent/caregiver *supports* the child's *pretending* (to be someone else; to do something else; that an object is something else; that something else is happening). Parent/caregiver may enter into the pretend play as well.	2	Matt asks Sabrina to make coffee, but she makes pizza instead in her toy kitchen on the other side of the room. Matt encourages symbolic play several times throughout the observation but does not demonstrate pretense behavior himself. He might have encouraged her to engage for longer periods by pretending.
14. Parent/caregiver *supports* or encourages the child to *incorporate* objects or other people into play in *unconventional or variable* ways.	2	Matt was too concerned with Sabrina's safety to let her explore what to do with the bin. He might have encouraged her to engage for longer periods through unconventional use of objects or people.
15. Parent/caregiver adheres to *consistent, reasonable, and clear boundaries or rules.* Rules do not change unexpectedly.	3	Matt provides clear directions in clear situations.
16. Parent/caregiver *verbally praises* the child for a desired and appropriate behavior during play interaction.	1	Not evident but may partially be a reflection of the difficulty the two have in becoming engaged for longer periods of time.
Average score	**Sum of column scores/16 or number of items scored, excluding items scored NA**	**21/16 = 1.3**

SCORING REASONING

- *Caregiver and protector:* Matt is engaged in the joint play experience; however, he does not support Sabrina's ability to focus on any play activity for more than a few minutes (see Items 1, 2, and 5). Matt provided clear boundaries and supported Sabrina's sense of safety during the joint play experience (see Items 6 and 15).
- *Nurturer:* Matt's affect is fairly neutral, and he did not provide praise throughout the joint play experience (see Items 4 and 16).
- *Educator and learner:* There was little support of self-exploration, learning, or creativity in play activities (see Items 3, 7, 8, 9, 10, 11, 12, 13, and 14). Matt supported Sabrina's incorporating new ideas or objects into play, negotiation skills, and pretend play. He provided suggestions based on Sabrina's preferences or how she reacted to his previous suggestions. This may be based on self-learning, observing, and self-correction.

SUGGESTIONS FOR INTERVENTION

Sabrina seemed to have difficulty becoming totally engaged in any activity; she transitioned very rapidly between activities. Help Matt develop strategies to extend play activities. If that does not help Sabrina become more engaged, it may be useful to assess Sabrina with the Test of Playfulness as the basis for setting up goals to promote Sabrina's playfulness and play skills.

Michael and Jennifer

Michael is age 35 years and married. He works as a high school teacher. **Jennifer** is age 2 years, 10 months, and the oldest of two children. Jennifer attends daycare 3 days a week and spends other days at home with her mother and baby brother. Jennifer's parents contacted an early intervention occupational therapist to discuss her development. They wanted to make sure they provided Jennifer with an engaging and conducive environment, especially because she spends 2 weekdays at home with her mother and baby brother. Jennifer reached developmental milestones on time. Her preferred language is English.

JOINT PLAY OBSERVATION

Michael and Jennifer were observed playing at home in a space they usually play in. There was constant background noise. They played on the floor in front of a small dollhouse surrounded by small dolls; both played with the dolls. Jennifer described each doll, giving names to each. Michael asked Jennifer continuous questions about the doll's names and clothes. Jennifer tried putting clothes and other accessories on the dolls independently but often asked Michael for help.

Michael asked Jennifer whether they were going to go shopping, but Jennifer continued putting clothes and accessories on and taking them off the dolls. She began putting the dolls into the dollhouse, naming each and giving each an accessory and a bed. She said she was creating a sleepover for the dolls. Michael asked questions of each doll. Jennifer said she wanted the dolls to sleep for 5 minutes. Michael asked her to count to five and then wake them up. Jennifer pointed to or picked up each doll, speaking for them. Jennifer said the dolls need more sleep, but Michael continued to ask to wake them up. Michael began looking around and asking more questions about the dolls and their accessories. He continued to ask questions about the names of the dolls and pretended one doll was playing with another doll. Jennifer began removing clothes from the dolls and switching clothing from one to another. She often asked Michael for help with the dolls' clothing. Jennifer thanked Michael every time he helped her. She pretended to speak for the dolls and picked up each doll when they were "talking." Michael responded as though the dolls were speaking to him. Jennifer continued trying to change the clothes of each doll, and Michael watched as she tried, offering help when needed. Scoring for Michael and Jennifer is shown in Table 5.4.

TABLE 5.4. Michael and Jennifer PC–SCP Scoring

Dyad (#): Michael and Jennifer **Age:** **Rater:** **In Out Video Live (Circle)**	**Scale** **NA = not applicable** **0 = low** **1 = mild** **2 = moderate** **3 = high**	
Items	**Score**	**Comments**
1. Parent/caregiver is *actively supporting* the child's engagement in free play.	3	Examples of active support of child's engagement in free play: "There are multiple small dolls in front of them, and both are playing with the dolls. Jennifer is describing each doll and giving names to each doll. Michael asks questions about the doll's names and clothes." Michael sometimes tries to change the direction of the play (e.g., asks if they are going shopping) but does not persist when Jennifer does not pick up his suggestion.
2. Parent/caregiver supports the child's engagement in the activity *for the process* rather than primarily for the end product (building, assembling, and "getting the job done").	3	Michael promotes Jennifer's engagement based on her play interests in a clear and consistent manner. For example, "He continues to ask questions about the names of the dolls and pretends one doll is playing with another doll."
3. Parent/caregiver *helps* the child *overcome barriers or obstacles* to persist with the activity.	2	Jennifer feels comfortable asking Michael for help; he assists her effortlessly without affecting the continuation of the play.
4. Parent/caregiver demonstrates *positive affect* during play.	2	Seems neutral although he is engaged. This type of play does not call for laughter or overt signs of joy.
5. Parent/caregiver *supports* the child in *decision making*.	3	Michael lets Jennifer take the lead in joint play and asks her attuned questions that show that he lets her make decisions about the direction of play.
6. Parent/caregiver *provides a sense of safety* during play, so the child will feel sufficiently safe (emotionally and physically) to keep playing (e.g., selecting toys, coming up with ideas, making modifications, feeling safe to make choices or move around).	3	Jennifer seems to feel safe playing, asking for help, and answering her dad's questions.
7. Parent/caregiver *supports* the child's *modifications* or their needs to *modify* the activity to maintain the challenge or make it more fun.	3	Michael spontaneously and effortlessly supports several modifications that Jennifer makes.
8. Parent/caregiver *supports the child in interacting with objects* during play.	3	Continuous support of Jennifer's interaction with the dolls and their clothing and accessories. He might have done a little more to help her master putting on or taking off the dolls' clothing.

(Continued)

TABLE 5.4. Michael and Jennifer PC–SCP Scoring *(Cont.)*

Items	Score	Comments
9. Parent/caregiver *supports* the child's *transition* from one activity to the other when the first no longer evolves or suits the child's preferences or needs or supports the child to remain with an activity that is meeting the child's needs.	3	Michael senses that Jennifer enjoys playing with the dolls and is interested, and the transitions are in the form of questions that keep them both engaged and attuned to one another.
10. Parent/caregiver *supports* the child's *negotiations* to have their desires met in a suitable, respectful, and age-appropriate manner.	3	There are verbal exchanges that are clear and support the continuation of the joint play interaction.
11. Parent/caregiver *supports* the child's needs in *social play*.	3	Clear synchrony.
12. Parent/caregiver *supports* the child's engagement in playful *mischief, clowning*, or *joking*, or the parent/caregiver incorporates playful *mischief, clowning*, or *joking* during play.	2	Sophisticated mischief: "Michael asked her to count to five and then wake them up. Jennifer pointed to or picked up each doll, speaking for them. Jennifer said the dolls need more sleep, but Michael continued to ask to wake them up."
13. Parent/caregiver *supports* the child's *pretending* (to be someone else; to do something else; that an object is something else; that something else is happening). Parent/caregiver may enter into the pretend play as well.	3	There is a continuous support of pretend play.
14. Parent/caregiver *supports* or encourages the child to *incorporate* objects or other people into play in *unconventional or variable* ways.	2	Encourages incorporating new ideas (e.g., naming the dolls, shopping, waking up the dolls).
15. Parent/caregiver adheres to *consistent, reasonable, and clear boundaries or rules*. Rules do not change unexpectedly.	3	The boundaries are clear, and there is no negotiation around them.
16. Parent/caregiver *verbally praises* the child for a desired and appropriate behavior during play interaction.	NA	Not evident, but praise should always be genuine and genuinely needed in a play situation—and that is not the case here.
Average score	**Sum of column scores/16 or number of items scored, excluding items scored NA**	**42/15 = 2.8**

SCORING REASONING

- *Caregiver and protector:* Michael's presence in the joint play experience is evident. He consistently supported process-oriented behavior and encouraged Jennifer to make decisions and acknowledged her choices (see Items 1, 2, and 5). Michael provided a physically and emotionally safe environment where Jennifer played and explored ideas, objects, and space (see Items 6 and 15).
- *Nurturer:* Jennifer was very engaged in pretend play; although no affection or praise were noted, these might have been disruptive to the play (see Items 4 and 16).
- *Educator and learner:* Michael supported child-directed play, facilitating Jennifer's pretend play rather than engaging in direct teaching (see Items 3, 7, 8, 9, 10, 11, 12, 13, and 14). Michael appeared to be attuned to Jennifer's needs and preferences during play.

SUGGESTIONS FOR INTERVENTION

In this example, the parent provided suitable support, and the only point of feedback is to discuss the benefits of incorporating praise and affection into play interactions as appropriate.

Kelly and James

Kelly is age 42 years and married. She works full-time in information technology for a software company. **James,** age 9 years, 5 months, is the youngest of her three children. James is bilingual and speaks Russian and English. He attends a private elementary school and is reported to be doing well academically. Kelly contacted an occupational therapist whom she had known because one of her older children received childhood occupational therapy services. Kelly was worried that James was spending too much time on computer games, and it is more challenging for her to interact with him.

JOINT PLAY OBSERVATION

Kelly and James were observed playing at home, sitting at the dining room table with a block design game placed in the middle of the table. Kelly adjusted herself in her seat, and James also adjusted his posture (observer's note: possibly mirroring Kelly's movements), then leaned forward to put blocks on the game board. Kelly was speaking to a family member standing in the kitchen, and then she looked back in James's direction. Kelly and James conversed about the rules while both looking toward the game. When James put a block on the board, Kelly made an "uh-uh " sound, and James asked, "No?" James picked up another piece and prepared to place it on the board. Kelly spoke while James looked at the model picture and placed more pieces on the board. James explained why he thought the pieces fit where he put them. Kelly said, "Okay." Kelly suggested that James put a certain piece on the board. James responded with a question, and Kelly answered, "Mm-hm." Then James put down more blocks. Both James and Kelly were leaning toward one another. James placed the final block and looked toward Kelly, who lifted the game up off the table.

Kelly picked a new model card and placed it in front of James. James picked a block and tried to figure out where to place it. He looked at Kelly, but she looked the other way at her phone. Then she picked up a block and asked James to place it. Now James held two blocks. He tried to see where they both fit, based on the model picture. James was looking down interacting with the game, speaking softly to himself or possibly to Kelly. James picked a new card and asked Kelly if he should try that one. Kelly responded, "Sure, why not?" Then Kelly took the card from James and looked at it. Talking about the game, Kelly told James he should try matching more blocks until he matched the design. James leaned on the table, laying his head on his hands as if he was giving up. He continued playing in that position. Kelly counted the pieces on the board. While she was counting, James dropped a piece on the floor and picked it up. Kelly was verifying that James's pieces were correct (observer's note: "maybe made James nervous or just distracted, leading to the piece slipping out of his hand"). James tried to place another piece and then said, "This is boring. I want to do something else." Kelly responded, "But we should finish this first." James got up, saying he was looking for a different game. Scoring for Kelly and James is shown in Table 5.5.

TABLE 5.5. Kelly and James PC–SCP Scoring

Dyad (#): Kelly and James **Age:** **Rater:** **In** **Out** **Video** **Live** **(Circle)**	**Scale** **NA = not applicable** **0 = low** **1 = mild** **2 = moderate** **3 = high**	
Items	**Score**	**Comments**
1. Parent/caregiver is *actively supporting* the child's engagement in free play.	1	Kelly is not fully engaged or focused on James's needs in play. For example, Kelly is speaking to a family member. James looks at Kelly, but she looks the other way at her phone.
2. Parent/caregiver supports the child's engagement in the activity *for the process* rather than primarily for the end product (building, assembling, and "getting the job done").	1	The focus is on putting the model together and less on the process.
3. Parent/caregiver *helps* the child *overcome barriers or obstacles* to persist with the activity.	1	James's main obstacle is putting together the model, and eventually he gets bored. Kelly does not seem to identify that barrier on time.
4. Parent/caregiver demonstrates *positive affect* during play.	1	Neutral affect, but that is likely what this game calls for.
5. Parent/caregiver *supports* the child in *decision-making*.	2	Kelly is clearly trying to assist James in deciding what to do and promote shared decision making. However, sometimes her actions lack attunement.
6. Parent/caregiver *provides a sense of safety* during play, so the child will feel sufficiently safe (emotionally and physically) to keep playing (e.g., selecting toys, coming up with ideas, making modifications, feeling safe to make choices or move around).	1	James looks at Kelly for validation or reassurance, which may reflect a lower sense of emotional safety; however, Kelly does not capture those signals.
7. Parent/caregiver *supports* the child's *modifications* or their needs to *modify* the activity to maintain the challenge or make it more fun.	NA	Because this is a structured game, it does not really call for modification, and it seems difficult enough as it is. Silly modifications would not be appropriate for a child of this age.
8. Parent/caregiver *supports the child in interacting with objects* during play.	2	There was a continuous effort to assist James to place pieces or blocks in the correct place or position.
9. Parent/caregiver *supports* the child's *transition* from one activity to the other when the first no longer evolves or suits the child's preferences or needs or supports the child to remain with an activity that is meeting the child's needs.	0	James got bored (frustrated), and there was no support for transitioning between play activities.
10. Parent/caregiver *supports* the child's *negotiations* to have their desires met in a suitable, respectful, and age-appropriate manner.	1	Simple verbal exchanges.

(Continued)

TABLE 5.5. Kelly and James PC–SCP Scoring *(Cont.)*

Items	Score	Comments
11. Parent/caregiver *supports* the child's needs in *social play*.	2	There was evident back-and-forth verbal and nonverbal interaction. (Both James and Kelly leaned their bodies toward the other. Indicates interest in playing together).
12. Parent/caregiver *supports* the child's engagement in playful *mischief, clowning*, or *joking*, or the parent/caregiver incorporates playful *mischief, clowning, or joking* during play.	NA	This is not an activity that calls for mischief or clowning.
13. Parent/caregiver *supports* the child's *pretending* (to be someone else; to do something else; that an object is something else; that something else is happening). Parent/caregiver may enter into the pretend play as well.	NA	This is not an activity that calls for pretense. James is too old for much pretending in this contexts
14. Parent/caregiver *supports* and/or encourages the child in *incorporating* objects or other people into play in *unconventional or variable* ways.	NA	This is not an activity that calls for using objects unconventionally.
15. Parent/caregiver adheres to *consistent, reasonable, and clear boundaries or rules.* Rules do not change unexpectedly.	2	They discussed rules at the beginning; it seems like the setup is clear to both.
16. Parent/caregiver *verbally praises* the child for a desired and appropriate behavior during play interaction.	1	Minimal positive feedback.
Average score	**Sum of column scores/16 or number of items scored, excluding items scored NA**	**15/12 = 1.25**

SCORING REASONING

- *Caregiver and protector:* Kelly's support of James's engagement in process-oriented play is low; however, she does encourage him to make decisions during play (see Items 1, 2, and 5). Kelly let James explain the rules, which created a sense of safety and is age appropriate (see Items 6 and 15).
- *Nurturer:* Kelly's affect was neutral; she may need to provide more positive feedback to her son (see Items 4 and 16).
- *Educator and learner:* Kelly supports James's use of objects while assembling the model using direct cues (indicating where to place a block). She also encourages their engagement in social play. Other aspects of playfulness were not supported, but these may not be part of the kind of play in which they were engaging. During middle childhood, joint play often consists of board games and can lead to conversations between a parent and child that extend over the play interaction (see Items 3, 7, 8, 9, 10, 11, 12, 13, and 14). There was no evidence of self-correction or reflection.

SUGGESTIONS FOR INTERVENTION

- Discuss the role of play, playfulness, and joint play during middle childhood and ways to use joint play as an opportunity to continue psychosocial development.
- Encourage Kelly and James to find common interests in play and leisure that they can engage in and make a fun experience.

The co-occupation experience of joint play manifests in different ways. Parent or caregiver support of their child's playfulness is shaped by their own personal thoughts and feelings as well as their child's play preferences, needs, and responses. Each parent or caregiver displays a different profile of very supportive and less supportive behaviors. Occupational therapy practitioners can capitalize on the cluster of co-occupation behaviors to further guide parent or caregiver joint play experiences.

6

Use of the PC–SCP in School Settings

Performance and engagement in play occupations are crucial to a child's development of identity, their perception of competence, and their overall health and wellness, regardless of whether they have a disability (American Occupational Therapy Association [AOTA], 2012, 2020; Laverdure & Beisbier, 2021). Moreover, there is a positive correlation between activity of daily living (ADL) performance, play and leisure performance, quality of life, and future employment outcomes among children and youth (Pierucci et al., 2015). Laverdure and Beisbier's (2021) systematic review revealed that engaging children and youth with disabilities in ADLs, play, and leisure while providing feedback on their performance and offering caregivers guidance by coaching them can improve occupational performance and participation in play and leisure.

This chapter focuses on the occupation of play in school settings. Although education is a student's primary occupation, there are many opportunities for students to engage in play activities in the context of school (AOTA, 2012, 2020; Frolek Clark & Ponsolle-Mays, 2019). School provides a social context in which the child, fulfilling their role as a student, interacts with peers and adults in group and individualized activities. In this context, opportunities for play exist in a variety of settings, such as on a school bus traveling to and from school, during recess, during physical education, in clubs that meet before or after school, in free play, and in play-based educational programs (AOTA, 2012, 2020; Frolek Clark & Ponsolle-Mays, 2019).

Laws and Regulations That Support Play in School Settings

Several federal, state, and local laws and regulations support play in the school system. The federally mandated Individuals With Disabilities Education Improvement Act of 2004 (IDEA; P. L. 108-446) and Every Student Succeeds Act (ESSA; 2015, P. L. 114-195) aim to ensure equal opportunities for all students, regardless of whether they have a disability. This includes access to play, recess, and leisure pursuits. The Americans With Disabilities Act of 1990 (ADA; P. L. 101-336) and Section 504 of the Rehabilitation Act of 1973 (P. L. 93-112) prohibit discrimination based on disability, thereby paving the way for accommodations and modifications to be made to environments and activities to create more opportunities for play (U.S. Department of Health and Human Services, 2006). In addition, Article 31 of the United Nations Convention on the Rights of the Child stipulates that children have the right to play and have fun in ways that they want to. It also states that governments should ensure that play is easy for children to participate in regardless of whether they have a disability (UNICEF, n.d.).

Play and Dynamic Systems Theory

Play "is a complex and multidimensional phenomenon that is shaped by sociocultural factors" (AOTA, 2020, p. 81). Play is affected by many variables, such as familial culture, the culture of the school system, student factors, school-based personnel factors, and the daily activities in which the student is expected to participate (Frolek Clark

& Ponselle-Mays, 2019). In this section, we describe a theoretical framework, Bronfenbrenner's (1983) Ecological Systems Theory (EST) of human development, which is rooted in dynamic systems theory, and apply it to school play.

Bronfenbrenner's (1983) EST is a dynamic systems theory that considers the interplay of biological, psychological, and social sciences and how all systems affect one another and the individual. Bronfenbrenner identified five systems that relate to one another and to the child: the microsystem, mesosystem, exosystem, macrosystem, and chronosystem.

MICROSYSTEM

The *microsystem* includes the child's personality, beliefs, and temperament, as well as the people with whom a child has daily, face-to-face contact. It may include family members and educators (Bronfenbrenner, 1983). An example of a microsystem that affects play and social participation is a child's emotional state. Consider Joe, age 7 years, who is upset that his father forgot to give him money for today's book fair. Joe would typically play with his classmates during recess; however, today his emotional state interferes with his ability to focus on anything but the book fair. Instead of playing during recess, he sits on a bench by himself and ruminates.

MESOSYSTEM

The *mesosystem* is made up of links between multiple microsystems in a child's life (Bronfenbrenner, 1983). The classroom, classmates, and educators create a microsystem for an individual student. The school, broader student body, and the school staff make up a mesosystem for the student (Bronfenbrenner, 1983). If we use the case of Joe, an example of a mesosystem that affects Joe's play and social participation on the playground is his relationship with Mrs. P., the recess aide. Mrs. P. gives Joe the job of distributing the basketballs during recess, thereby supporting his occupational engagement. Joe accepts this job because he has a trusting and respectful relationship with Mrs. P.

EXOSYSTEM

The *exosystem* is like the mesosystem; however, in the exosystem, at least one of the microsystems does not contain the student at the center of it. Although the student is not at the center of this system, they may be affected by things that occur within it (Bronfenbrenner, 1983). Considering the case of Joe again, an example of an exosystem that affects his occupational engagement is the school's policy on recess participation. All students are expected to participate in recess and not sit on the bench. This policy contributed to the recess aide, Mrs. P., approaching Joe on the bench and offering him a way to participate, despite his emotional state, thereby supporting his occupational engagement.

MACROSYSTEM

The *macrosystem* represents culture and societal structures. In the case of Joe, an example of a macrosystem affecting his participation in play is his teacher's cultural views on her role in supporting play versus education. If Joe's teacher values education highly and does not value the role that play has in development, Joe will not be provided with opportunities to engage in the occupation of play during the day.

CHRONOSYSTEM

The *chronosystem* addresses the concept of time. It includes the student's aging and maturation and the time in which they live and develop (Bronfenbrenner, 1983). The SARS-CoV-2 virus (COVID-19) pandemic is an example of a chronosystem that affected countless children's play opportunities and behaviors. Consider what play looked like before the pandemic, both in and out of the context of the school building, and what it looks like now. Around the world, students who received their education in a school building prepandemic suddenly received their education remotely. This prevented many children from engaging in cooperative play with peers. As education returned to the school building, mask mandates affected students' abilities to receive social, visual, and, in some cases, auditory cues from their play partners. This is an example of how a chronosystem can have a profound impact on a student's ability to develop and maintain play behaviors.

Teachers and School-Based Support Personnel as Play Partners

Historically, play therapy, an evidence-based form of child psychotherapy, has been practiced and delivered by clinical psychologists with the intention of supporting and assisting children with socioemotional problems through the medium of play (Flasch et al., 2017; Landreth, 2012; Lin & Bratton, 2015; Pereira & Smith-Adcock, 2013; Ray et al., 2015; Shin & Gonzalez, 2018). This child-centered approach uses play as a means to an end, with the end being the child's social, emotional, and psychological functioning and adjustment. Play is the medium or means through which a child may explore underlying social and emotional conflicts.

An example of play therapy as a means rather than an end is illustrated by Aisha, a second grader who is experiencing bullying on the school bus. Aisha's school-based registered play therapist, a social worker credentialed in play therapy, provided her with a variety of toys, dolls, and art and crafts supplies because child-centered play therapy is built on the belief that the child will innately know what materials they need to work through social–emotional challenges they might be experiencing. Aisha selected crayons and paper and drew a picture of herself on the school bus on the day when she was bullied. With encouragement from the play therapist, she was then able to use the dolls to act out a situation in which she successfully navigated the bus ride without a bullying incident.

Play-based interventions may be used by occupational therapy practitioners; however, these interventions have limited implementation in school-based practice (Waldman-Levi & Weintraub, 2015). Fabrizi et al. (2016) conducted a study to determine whether an occupational therapist–led play group provided once per week for 8 weeks influenced the playfulness of children with special needs ages 15 months to 3 years and the responsiveness of their caregivers. They concluded that all children participating in the study benefited from the occupational therapy playgroup intervention and exhibited an increase in playful behavior after the intervention. Moreover, caregiver participation in community-based playgroups supports the transition from the community to the preschool (Fabrizi et al., 2016). In an interdisciplinary study, Bundy et al. (2015) looked at the playfulness of children on a playground after an occupational therapy intervention and stakeholder education. The authors highlighted the distinct value of occupational therapists as play and collaboration experts and suggested that occupational therapy practitioners are distinctly prepared to work with educators and other stakeholders to problem-solve playground challenges and support child success (Bundy et al., 2015; Sterman et al., 2020).

Although trained school-based play therapists may directly intervene with students to address the root causes of psychological, social, and emotional challenges, school-based caretakers, such as related service providers, recess aides, teachers, and classroom staff, can support a student's success as they engage in play-based activities that support learning (Frolek Clark & Ponselle-Mays, 2019). Aisha's teacher, Mrs. Lee, provided structure for group work by creating group ground rules that encourage respectful group behavior. Mrs. Lee posted the group ground rules where all students could see them and routinely monitored the groups to make sure that all members were treated fairly and that no bullying occurred.

Some exosystem and macrosystem challenges that school-based caretakers encounter and that cause a barrier to supporting students' play include lack of (1) assessments identifying areas in which caretakers need assistance to facilitate play (Ebrahim et al., 2012; Shin & Gonzalez, 2018), (2) training and education in group dynamics, and (3) time dedicated to supporting student play. At the exosystem level, education and training in the facilitation of play might influence policy development, such as schoolwide adoption of increased recess time. At the macrosystem level, education and training would influence stakeholders' beliefs about the importance of play, thereby supporting policy changes.

Interdisciplinary collaboration is crucial when supporting students' play in the school context (AOTA, 2020; Shepherd et al., 2019). Such collaboration increases the likelihood of improved student outcomes by cooperatively collaborating on shared student goals, increasing consistent use of strategies across multiple contexts, and decreasing redundancies in intervention (Shepherd et al., 2019).

As related service providers, occupational therapy practitioners regard play as a primary occupation of childhood (AOTA, 2016). Consequently, they work collaboratively with medical providers, educators, and other health professionals to design inclusive programs that promote play on playgrounds, as well as during curricular and extracurricular pursuits (AOTA, 2016). In the next section, we explore the role of the occupational therapist in school-based play assessment and intervention.

Role of the Occupational Therapist in School-Based Play Assessment and Intervention

Approximately 23% of occupational therapists and 19% of occupational therapy assistants work in early intervention and school settings (AOTA, 2019). They support individual students, groups of students, populations of children within classrooms, and whole-school programming (AOTA, 2016). Occupational therapy practitioners are trained to support all students in their academic and nonacademic pursuits, including, but not limited to, math, literacy, social skills, behavior management, recess, participation in sports, self-help skills, and transportation (AOTA, 2016). Occupational therapy practitioners focus on students' strengths as they design and implement services to improve inclusion and accessibility for all students in the school context (AOTA, 2016). They use their expertise to enhance student participation in occupations and provide interventions on behalf of the students by providing resources and building the capacity of families, caregivers, and education staff through targeted interventions focusing on engagement in daily living activities, social participation, education, play, and leisure (AOTA, 2020).

The occupational therapy process includes assessment and evaluation, intervention, and adaptation of tasks and the environment to support play (AOTA, 2020). Several assessments enable occupational therapists to assess aspects of children's play and playfulness. The Test of Playfulness and Test of Environmental Supportiveness (Skard & Bundy, 2008) and the Knox Preschool Play Scale (Knox, 2008) are primarily used with children. However, these assessments do not enable the assessment of play from a mesosystem perspective (e.g., how teachers, aides, or paraprofessionals support children's engagement in play and being playful). Using a valid and reliable assessment of teachers' and caregivers' support, such as the Parent/Caregiver's Support of Children's Playfulness (PC–SCP), can lead to the development and implementation of play-based interventions tailored to the needs of children in school settings, creating a better fit between the child and their environment or, in Bronfenbrenner's (1983) EST language, among the microsystem (child), mesosystem (classmates, teachers, play opportunities), and exosystem (play settings, administration). Moreover, technology may play a role in the occupational therapy process because it can be very motivating for young students (Garfinkel & Minard, 2021). As part of a positive behavioral support system in the schools, students can earn motivating play- and technology-based rewards that support desired behaviors (Garfinkel & Minard, 2021), thereby using play occupations as a means rather than an end or goal.

The following case study illustrates PC–SCP scoring based on observing a joint play interaction between a school-based caretaker and a student to exemplify opportunities to assess and promote play in a school setting.

Diane and Glenn

Diane is age 50 years and employed as a one-to-one aide for **Glenn** in a public elementary school. Glenn is age 5 years, 6 months, and is on the autism spectrum. Diane and Glenn were observed engaging in a play-based activity in a space within the classroom that is typically used during indoor recess. Glenn's preferred language is English, and he attends full-day kindergarten 5 days a week. Glenn is an only child who spends evenings and weekends at home with his mother and father.

JOINT PLAY OBSERVATION

Diane and Glenn are engaged in a play activity using Legos at a table in the back of the classroom during recess. There is constant loud background noise, and several of Glenn's classmates approach Diane, wanting to talk to her. Diane asks Glenn what he is building. He says a car. Diane asks Glenn whether she should build a car or an airplane. Glenn says a car so that they can race. Diane tells Glenn that she loves to watch race cars on TV. Glenn tells Diane about his favorite type of race car. Diane divides her attention between listening to Glenn and fielding questions from a teacher who enters the room to collect supplies. Although Glenn started off initiating conversation about the Legos and cars, he later engaged more in solitary play, whereas Diane's attention was pulled to the teacher. When Diane finished answering the teacher's questions, she asked Glenn if he had four wheels for his car. Glenn said "Yes," and he took his finished car and pretended he was on a racetrack, guiding the car along the edge of the table. Glenn asked Diane if they could race. Diane said, "In a minute," as she put a bandage on her finger. When she was done with the bandage, she continued to build her own car. Glenn continued to play alone with his car until Diane finished her car and began to pretend to drive her car around the same race track that Glenn was driving on. Glenn started to crash his car into Diane's aggressively. She told him that he almost pinched her finger and that it was not nice to crash cars. Glenn became upset and said, "Race cars crash." He tried to roll his car over, but the wheels fell off his car. He stomped his feet and yelled, "See what you made me do?" Diane said that she would not play with him until he played nicely. Glenn threw his car on the floor and said, "I hate Legos." Scoring for Diane and Glenn is shown in Table 6.1.

TABLE 6.1. Diane and Glenn PC–SCP Scoring

Dyad (#): Diane and Glenn **Age:** **Rater:** **In** **Out** **Video** **Live** **(Circle)**		**Quality Scale** **NA = not applicable** **0 = low** **1 = mild** **2 = moderate** **3 = high**
Items	**Score**	**Comments**
1. Parent/caregiver is *actively supporting* the child's engagement in free play.	2	Diane asks Glenn about his race car. She asks Glenn what she should build with the Legos. Diane tells Glenn that she likes to watch race cars on TV. However, Diane is often distracted by other students in the classroom, dividing her attention between Glenn and his classmates. Diane is not attentive to Glenn's need for continual engagement with her. She tells him he cannot play if he continues to play aggressively.
2. Parent/caregiver supports the child's engagement in the activity *for the process* rather than primarily for the end product (building, assembling, and "getting the job done").	1	Diane begins playing with Glenn, and then her attention is pulled to other students in the classroom, leaving Glenn to play by himself. Diane reengages with Glenn once he has finished making his Lego car, asking Glenn if he has wheels for his car and then telling him that he is playing incorrectly by crashing it. Her engagement seems to be disrupted and task oriented.

(Continued)

TABLE 6.1. Diane and Glenn PC–SCP Scoring *(Cont.)*

Items	Score	Comments
3. Parent/caregiver *helps* the child *overcome barriers or obstacles* to persist with the activity.	0	After Diane told Glenn that he was playing too aggressively, Glenn became upset. Diane did not help him manage his emotions, thereby effectively ending the play experience.
4. Parent/caregiver demonstrates *positive affect* during play.	1	Diane began the play activity with a positive affect; however, it became negative once Glenn began crashing his car into her car.
5. Parent/caregiver *supports* the child in *decision making*.	0	Not evident.
6. Parent/caregiver *provides a sense of safety* during play, so the child will feel sufficiently safe (emotionally and physically) to keep playing (e.g., selecting toys, coming up with ideas, making modifications, feeling safe to make choices or move around).	0	Diane did not support a sense of safety; rather, she stopped the play when Glenn began playing unsafely.
7. Parent/caregiver *supports* child's *modifications* or their needs to *modify* the activity to maintain the challenge or make it more fun.	0	Not evident.
8. Parent/caregiver *supports the child in interacting with objects* during play.	1	Diane supported Glenn's building endeavors but then stopped Glenn from pretend play.
9. Parent/caregiver *supports* the child's *transition* from one activity to the other when the first no longer evolves or suits the child's preferences or needs or supports the child to remain with an activity that is meeting the child's needs.	0	Diane did not support Glenn's transition away from the Legos. She stopped the activity, and when Glenn walked away, she did not help him to end the activity positively.
10. Parent/caregiver *supports* the child's *negotiations* to have their desires met in a suitable, respectful, and age-appropriate manner.	0	Diane told Glenn what her expectations were for racing the car. When Glenn did not adhere to the instructions, she did not facilitate negotiation skills.
11. Parent/caregiver *supports* the child's needs in *social play*.	1	Diane's attention was pulled from Glenn as other students approached her during recess. She did not set boundaries with the other students, allowing them to interrupt her play with Glenn. Because she was continually distracted by Glenn's classmates, she was not available to him (for social play) for a good portion of the activity.
12. Parent/caregiver *supports* the child's engagement in playful *mischief, clowning*, or *joking*, or the parent/caregiver incorporates playful *mischief, clowning*, or *joking* during play.	1	When Glenn became mischievous, crashing and rolling his car, Diane stopped the play. This effectively stopped Glenn's attempt at being mischievous.
13. Parent/caregiver *supports* the child's *pretending* (to be someone else; to do something else; that an object is something else; that something else is happening). Parent/caregiver may enter into the pretend play as well.	2	Diane encouraged Glenn to make the Legos into a race car. Once the car was built, however, she did not support Glenn's pretending that his race car was crashing.

(Continued)

TABLE 6.1. Diane and Glenn PC–SCP Scoring *(Cont.)*

Items	Score	Comments
14. Parent/caregiver *supports* or encourages the child to *incorporate* objects or other people into play in *unconventional or variable* ways.	0	Not evident.
15. Parent/caregiver adheres to *consistent, reasonable, and clear boundaries or rules.* Rules do not change unexpectedly.	1	Diane was inconsistent. She began the Lego activity, encouraging Glenn to be creative. When Glenn sought her attention, she was not available because she was tending to other students. Diane did not set boundaries with the other students, allowing them to interrupt the play experience for Glenn. Although she led Glenn to believe that they would pretend to race cars, she changed the rules by not allowing Glenn to play the way he wanted to with the race cars.
16. Parent/caregiver *verbally praises* the child for a desired and appropriate behavior during play interaction.	0	Not evident.
Average score	**Sum of column scores/16 or the number of items scored, excluding items scored NA**	**10/16 = 0.62**

SCORING REASONING

- *Caregiver and protector:* Diane's presence in the joint play experience was inconsistent. Initially, she supported Glenn's free play with the Legos; however, she allowed other students to distract her as she played with Glenn. She did not actively engage him in the play process (Item 2) and in fact stopped him from engaging when he played aggressively with the Lego car. Rather than helping him manage his emotions and behaviors, she stopped the game (see Items 1, 8, and 13). Diane inconsistently provided an emotionally safe environment where Glenn could play and explore ideas, objects, and space (see Items 6 and 15). Diane did not support Glenn in making decisions while playing or negotiating play themes or ideas (Item 5).
- *Nurturer:* Diane was not consistently engaged in pretend play, and no affection or praise were noted (see Items 4 and 16).
- *Educator and learner:* Diane did not support child-directed play. She scolded Glenn for not adhering to rules that she had yet to inform him about (no crashing cars). She could have instructed Glenn in how to play more safely with his Lego car (see Items 3, 7, 8, 9, 10, 11, 12, 13, and 14). Diane was not sensitive to Glenn's needs and preferences during play. She seems to be reactive, which may suggest that she needs to be more self-reflective.

SUGGESTIONS FOR INTERVENTION

- Glenn's one-to-one aide did not support Glenn's need for consistent attention and appropriate social play. She could benefit from consultation focused on providing consistent attention during social play and support to help him manage emotions and behaviors associated with pretend play. Direct stakeholder education and training may be used to provide feedback.
- There is a need for reinforcement of play-based strategies introduced during direct intervention to be carried over in natural environments when there are opportunities within the school context to apply play-based strategies.
- This case illustrates an opportunity for interprofessional collaboration in support of children with multiple needs. Through collaboration, stakeholders may support student playfulness through consistent facilitation, communication, and social participation, ultimately leading to an improved sense of self-efficacy and overall student health and wellness.

All children, regardless of ability or disability, are entitled to access play opportunities at school. These rights are supported by federal, state, and local laws and regulations. As illustrated in the case examples, play in school settings is affected by many variables, including familial and school culture, student factors, school-based personnel factors, and the types of available play. Occupational therapy practitioners working in schools have ample opportunities to support play through policy change, environmental modifications, and cultural and personal adaptations. Awareness of play's centrality to everyday life, assessments to guide intervention, and programmatic changes are key to supporting children's play.

7

Development and Psychometric Properties

The Parent/Caregiver Support of Children's Playfulness (PC–SCP) is based on literature describing child playfulness, adult playfulness, parent–child interaction, and play. In addition, well-established assessments served as inspiration, such as the Test of Playfulness (ToP; Skard & Bundy, 2008), the Test of Environmental Supportiveness (TOES; Skard & Bundy, 2008), and the Coding Interactive Behavior system (Feldman & Eidelman, 2005; Feldman et al., 2004; Feldman & Klein, 2003). See Waldman-Levi and Bundy (2016) for a detailed description of the literature supporting the PC–SCP.

Development of the PC–SCP

Creating the PC–SCP has been a rigorous, iterative, multistep process. This process will undoubtedly continue for some time as we gather additional data and learn more about this construct.

Originally, the PC–SCP consisted of 27 items, each scored in two areas: quality and frequency. In a pilot study, Waldman-Levi et al. (2017) examined preliminary psychometric properties of data gathered with the early version. Results provided evidence for criterion validity; mothers who supported their child's playfulness and exploration had more playful offspring. Although the pilot study had a small sample, the PC–SCP showed excellent evidence for internal consistency (ages 1–4 years, 8 months, quality $\alpha = .95$, frequency $\alpha = .85$; $N = 8$). We also examined interrater reliability using percentage of agreement; although it was acceptable for most children (i.e., ages 12 months–2 years, 60%–80%, $n = 4$; ages 3–5 years, 21%–72%, $n = 4$), the sample size was very small, and we felt the assessment required additional work.

On the basis of these preliminary results, a panel of expert pediatric occupational therapists examined PC–SCP item definitions while observing videos of infants and toddlers during joint play with their mothers. The review panel recommended removing some items because they were redundant. They also suggested items that should be scored only on quality (omitting frequency). The review panel's recommendations matched the list of items that had low interrater agreement. As a result, we eliminated 7 items (both quality and frequency) and, of the remaining items, chose to score frequency for only 10.

After these revisions, in additional studies (Waldman-Levi, Finzi-Dottan, & Cope, 2019; Waldman-Levi, Grinion, & Olson, 2019), we confirmed evidence for internal consistency of the overall test ($\alpha = .68$). We found that interrater reliability improved and was satisfactory. Agreement between raters ranged from 81% to 100%; the Cohen's κ of .611 ($p < .001$) was moderate.

Preliminary Studies of Psychometric Properties of Data Gathered With the PC–SCP

Early on, we conducted two exploratory factor analyses with principal-components factor extraction. In the first, which included both Quality and Frequency scale items, two factors emerged: Flow (item loading ranged from

.609 to .819) and Creative (item loading ranged from .450 to .810). In the second, which included only the Quality items, four factors emerged; the first accounted for 41.5% of the cumulative variance, the second for 53.0%, the third for 62.4%, and the fourth for 70.0%. Only the first and second factors had enough items with adequate loading to define them as constructs. The two factors used were (1) Flow, consisting of nine items of parent or caregiver behaviors that support engagement in play and frame the experience (item loading ranged from .609 to .819) and (2) Creativity, consisting of six items representing parent or caregiver behaviors that encourage creative and unconventional use of objects and ideas, fun-seeking behaviors, and positive outlook (item loading ranged from .450 to .810).

Criterion and Predictive Validity

We examined criterion validity in several cross-sectional studies examining associations with measures of child and adult playfulness, social–environmental supportiveness, and parental capacity to reflect on their child's behavior to guide their own behavior toward their child. The PC–SCP total score correlated with child playfulness as measured with the ToP (r = .33, p < .05), Quality and ToP (r = .27, p < .05), Frequency and ToP (r = .32, p < .05), and Flow and ToP (r = .41, p < .01; Waldman-Levi, Grinion, & Olson, 2019). The PC–SCP Quality scale significantly and positively correlated with the caregiver support items of the TOES (r = .37, p < .05; Waldman-Levi, Grinion, & Olson, 2019). The PC–SCP also correlated significantly with the Short Measure of Adult Playfulness (Proyer, 2012a; r = .87, p < .05; Waldman-Levi et al., 2017). The PC–SCP correlated with maternal capacity to reflect on the child's behavior as measured with the Parental Rumination-Reflection Questionnaire (PRQ; Trapnell & Campbell, 1999). More specifically, PC–SCP Quality and Frequency scales had low but statistically significant correlations with maternal reflective capacity (PC–SCP Quality and PRQ, r = .23, p = .05; PC–SCP Frequency and PRQ, r = .27, p < .05; Waldman-Levi, Grinion, & Olson, 2019).

For predictive validity, maternal reflective functioning as measured with the PRQ significantly predicted maternal supportive behavior during joint play. The general model was statistically significant but explained only 6% of the variance, R^2 = .27, F(1, 69) = 5.48, p < .05; β = .27, p < .05.

PC–SCP and Child Development

Findings from a longitudinal study of mothers and their infants at ages 6, 18, and 24 months showed that children's playfulness (ToP scores) significantly increased over time, whereas PC–SCP overall scores remained consistent: Quality, F(2, 40) = 1.02, p > .05; Frequency, F(1, 41) = 2.78, p > .05. Participants in this study had the following characteristics: There were no concerns about child development or relationship between parent and child; families lived in Israel and were non–English speaking; all children were firstborn; parents were heterosexual; most parents had a college-level education (Waldman-Levi, Bundy, & Shai, 2022).

Additional studies of parents and older children (Waldman-Levi, 2021; Waldman-Levi, Cope, & Olson, 2022; Waldman-Levi, Finzi-Dottan, & Cope, 2019; Waldman-Levi, Grinion, & Olson, 2019) confirmed findings that PC–SCP scores remain consistent even as children mature. Participants' characteristics in these studies were similar to those in the longitudinal study (Waldman-Levi et al., 2022) except that all were English speakers living in the United States. Table 7.1 displays the means and standard deviations for samples of mothers and fathers playing with their child across different age groups.

TABLE 7.1. Mothers' and Fathers' Support of Child's Playfulness Across Age Groups

PC–SCP Scale or Factor	*M* (*SD*)					
	Mothers and Children Ages 6 Mo (*n* = 42)	Mothers and Children Ages 18 Mo (*n* = 42)	Mothers and Children Ages 24 Mo (*n* = 42)	Mothers and Children Ages 12 Mo–6 Yr (*n* = 73)	Fathers and Children Ages 12 Mo–6 Yr (*n* = 55)	Mothers and Children Ages 6–11 Yr (*n* = 70)
Quality scale	2.58 (.33)	2.62 (.29)	2.67 (.33)	2.42 (.44)	2.04 (.50)	2.39 (.52)
Frequency scale	2.48 (.33)	2.71 (.61)	2.58 (.32)	2.46 (.34)	2.49 (.31)	—
Flow factor	—	—	—	2.65 (.60)	2.20 (.55)	2.52 (.50)
Creativity factor	—	—	—	2.03 (.65)	1.52 (.60)	2.04 (.74)

Note. — = not calculated.

Rasch Analysis

After preliminary studies that determined the final set of PC–SCP items, we conducted a Rasch analysis to determine whether the assessment represented a single construct. The Rasch model is a latent-trait psychometric model that transforms ordinal-level data into interval-level measures (Bond et al., 2020). The Rasch model is based on two straightforward assumptions: (1) that easier items (i.e., those that require less of the latent trait) are easier for all people and (2) that people with higher ability (i.e., more of the latent trait) will score higher on more difficult items than those with low ability. In terms of the PC–SCP, the latent trait is parental ability to support playfulness. Using the Rasch model, we can generate both item difficulty and person ability calibrations. For a full description of the Rasch model, please refer to Bond et al. (2020). Rasch modeling also provides several indicators of construct validity and reliability. We assessed these indicators and report them here.

Construct Validity

The Rasch model assumes that items and people form a unidimensional hierarchy—in other words, all items represent various levels of the latent trait (and are not affected by other, unrelated factors), and all people can be measured by using these items (Bond et al., 2020). Of course, this assumption rarely holds up perfectly in real-life measurement scenarios. Indicators provided by Winsteps (Version 5.4), the Rasch-specific software used in this analysis (Linacre, 2022), allowed us to examine the extent to which this assumption is (or is not) violated in the PC–SCP.

ITEM FIT

We examined the extent to which items adhere to the assumptions of the Rasch model by examining point-measure correlations and mean-square item fit statistics. Point-measure correlations indicate that the items align with the latent trait; all should be positive. Mean-squares represent the amount of noise introduced by unexpected responses (e.g., people with an overall low score who score remarkably high on more difficult items). The mean-square fit statistic for items represents the predictability in the pattern of responses (Bond et al., 2020; Linacre, 2022). The ideal value for mean-squares is 1.0; lower values indicate that items are too predictable, and higher values indicate that items are unpredictable. We considered values between 0.5 and 1.5 to indicate acceptable item fit. We examined both infit and outfit mean-squares. Infit mean-squares are weighted such that the responses given by people whose ability is close to the difficulty of the item have a larger impact on the value than people whose ability is far from the item difficulty. Outfit mean-squares are unweighted; as a result, they are more prone to be affected by outlying people or those with unexpected responses. We expected to see more variability in outfit mean-squares than in infit mean-squares. Because some items may fail to fit the model as a result of chance alone, we expected that no more than one item would fail to fit.

Table 7.2 contains item calibrations and fit statistics. All items had positive point-measure correlations. Only one item fell outside our desired criteria for goodness of fit. Item 15 ("parent/caregiver adheres to *consistent, reasonable, and clear boundaries or rules*; rules do not change unexpectedly") had an aberrant outfit mean-square (1.86). Infit statistics adhered to the model expectations. Further inspection of the data suggested that some parents who struggled to support their child's playfulness were still capable of setting and maintaining reasonable boundaries in play. Because this was the only item that failed to fit, and because infit was acceptable, we chose to retain this item. However, after inspection of the data and consideration of the scoring criteria, we modified the criteria for scores of 1 and 2 slightly to enable use of the full scale.

TABLE 7.2. Rasch Item Calibration and Fit Statistics

Item	Measure	*SE*	Point-Measure Correlation	Infit MnSq	Outfit MnSq
1	−1.86	0.16	0.50	1.13	0.83
2	−0.59	0.12	0.58	0.89	1.02
3	−1.11	0.14	0.59	0.76	0.73
4	0.4	0.11	0.69	0.71	0.81
5	−0.59	0.12	0.63	0.87	0.79
6	−0.34	0.12	0.68	0.81	0.78
7	0.45	0.11	0.62	1.38	1.32
8	−1.08	0.14	0.62	0.76	0.70
9	−0.2	0.12	0.62	1.11	1.06
10	−0.43	0.12	0.65	0.75	0.78
11	−0.62	0.13	0.68	0.74	0.65
12	2.34	0.13	0.68	1.12	1.15
13	1.63	0.11	0.68	1.31	1.26
14	1.66	0.11	0.73	1.16	1.15
15	−0.99	0.16	0.40	1.09	1.86
16	1.33	0.10	0.63	1.25	1.36

RATING SCALE ANALYSIS

In addition to providing data about item fit, Winsteps also allowed us to evaluate the extent to which rating scales within items fit the model. Because the majority of participating children and families had no concerns regarding any aspect of development or relationships, scores of 1 and 2 had been used only infrequently. Thus, in this preliminary Rasch analysis, we collapsed scores of 1 and 2, resulting in two rating scale structures: 1–2–3, which was used for Items 12 and 15, and 0–1–2–3, which was used for all other items.

We examined rating scale mean-square goodness-of-fit statistics using the same criteria as for items. We also examined Rasch–Andrich thresholds, which indicate the logit measure at which a person is equally likely to score in either of two adjacent categories. These categories should progress in an orderly fashion, such that the threshold between 0 and 1 is associated with a lower category measure than the threshold between 1 and 2, and so on.

Tables 7.3 and 7.4 contain the results of rating scale analyses. All Rasch–Andrich thresholds progressed as expected. Moreover, all rating scale categories fit the model for both scales except the two categories for the 1–2–3 rating scale. This category showed outfit statistics higher than 1.5, suggesting unexpected randomness. This category was used relatively infrequently, and infit statistics were perfect (1.00); therefore, although we considered this result acceptable at this stage of PC–SCP development, the structure of both these items should continue to be monitored, especially given changes to the scoring criteria.

TABLE 7.3. Rating Scale Goodness-of-Fit Statistics for Items With a 4-Point Scale

Category	Infit MnSq	Outfit MnSq	Rasch–Andrich Threshold[a]
0	1.26	1.29	
1	0.82	0.78	–1.27
2	1.00	0.87	–0.66
3	0.94	0.96	1.93

[a]Rasch–Andrich thresholds are reported for the adjacent category above each value (e.g., in the row labeled *2*, the Rasch–Andrich threshold is for Categories 1–2).

TABLE 7.4. Rating Scale Goodness-of-Fit Statistics for Items With a 3-Point Scale

Category	Infit MnSq	Outfit MnSq	Rasch–Andrich Threshold[a]
1	1.12	1.48	
2	1.00	1.64	–0.99
3	1.20	1.30	0.99

[a]Rasch–Andrich thresholds are reported for the adjacent category above each value (e.g., in the row labeled *2*, the Rasch–Andrich threshold is for Categories 1–2).

PERSON FIT

We also evaluated goodness-of-fit statistics for parents. In general, we expected more randomness from people than from items; therefore, we accepted mean-square fit statistics as long as they were less than 1.5. We sought 90% person fit to represent good adherence to the Rasch model. However, in this analysis, data from only 189/224 (84.4%) of parents fit the Rasch model. We will continue to monitor fit in further analyses. Such analyses will enable us to determine whether the characteristics of particular dyads lead them to use the PC–SCP items differently. If this is the case, it could lead to future changes to scoring.

ITEM SPREAD AND HIERARCHY

The Rasch model provides calibrations for item difficulties that can be visualized on a Wright map (see Figure 7.1). On the basis of this map, we examined the extent to which items followed a logical hierarchy, meaning that conceptually more difficult items are associated with more difficult item measures. We compared the item difficulties generated by the Rasch model for the PC–SCP with those generated by the model for ToP. We hypothesized that these would be

```
Raw Score     People          Items
      <More Playful>          <Requires More Playfulness>
      6    ######   +
                    |
                    |
                    |
                    |
                    |
      5       .##   +
                #   |
                .   |
                .  T|
                .   |
                    |
      4         #   +
                    |
          .######   |
                #   |
              ###   |
                .   |
      3    .#####  S+
                .   |
            .####   |
         .#######   |
                    |T   12 Mischief
               ##   |
      2      .###   +
             ####   |
            .####   |    13 Pretending        14 Unconventional
            .####  M|
              .##   |    16 Praise
            .####   |S
      1    ######   +
             ####   |
            .####   |
               ##   |    7  Modifications
            .####   |    4  Positive Affect
           ######   |
      0      ####  S+M
             ####   |    9  Transitions
              .##   |    6  Safety
              ###   |    10 Negotiations
               .#   |    11 Social Play       2  For Process        5  Decision Making
               .#   |
     -1         #   +    15 Rules             8  Objects
                    |S   3  Helps Overcome
                .   |
                   T|
                    |
                    |    1  Engagement
     -2             +
                    |
                    |T
                .   |
                    |
                    |
     -3             +
       <Less Playful>        <Requires Less Playfulness>
```

Figure 7.1 Wright map.

relatively similar; in other words, we expected that items that can only be accomplished by a more playful child could only be supported by a parent who is, themselves, highly playful. The difficulty of PC–SCP and ToP items is similar.

CONCLUSION

Taken collectively, these findings support the internal reliability and construct validity of the PC–SCP. Therefore, the PC–SCP can be a useful tool for occupational therapists and others working with parents and young children. As with all assessments, further research is warranted.

References

American Occupational Therapy Association. (2008). AOTA's societal statement on play. *American Journal of Occupational Therapy, 62,* 707–708. https://doi.org/10.5014/ajot.62.6.707

American Occupational Therapy Association. (2012). *Learning through play.* https://www.aota.org/~/media/Corporate/Files/AboutOT/consumers/Youth/Play/Learning%20Through%20Play%20tip%20sheet.pdfA

American Occupational Therapy Association. (2016). *Occupational therapy's role with school settings.* https://www.aota.org/-/media/Corporate/Files/AboutOT/Professionals/WhatIsOT/CY/Fact-Sheets/School%20Settings%20fact%20sheet.pdf

American Occupational Therapy Association. (2019). *2019 salary and workforce survey: Executive summary.* AOTA Press.

American Occupational Therapy Association. (2020). Occupational therapy practice framework: Domain and process (4th ed.). *American Journal of Occupational Therapy, 74*(Suppl. 2), 7412410010. https://doi.org/10.5014/ajot.2020.74S2001

Americans With Disabilities Act of 1990, Pub. L. No. 101-336, 42 U.S.C. §§ 12101–12213 (2000).

Association for Play Therapy. (2022). *Credentialing standards for the registered play therapist.* https://cdn.ymaws.com/www.a4pt.org/resource/resmgr/credentials/RPT_Standards.pdf

Auhuber, L., Vogel, M., Grafe, N., Kiess, W., & Poulain, T. (2019). Leisure activities of healthy children and adolescents. *International Journal of Environmental Research and Public Health, 16*(12), 2078. https://doi.org/10.3390/ijerph16122078

Barnett, L. A. (2007). The nature of playfulness in young adults. *Personality and Individual Differences, 43,* 949–958. https://doi.org/10.1016/j.paid.2007.02.018

Bazyk, S., Stalnaker, D., Llerena, M., Ekelman, B., & Bazyk, J. (2003). Play in Mayan children. *American Journal of Occupational Therapy, 57,* 273–283. https://doi.org/10.5014/ajot.57.3.273

Bekar, J. K., Fenning, R. M., Howland, M. A., Baucom, B. R., Moffitt, J., & Erath, S. A. (2015). Brief report: A pilot study of parent–child biobehavioral synchrony in autism spectrum disorder. *Journal of Autism and Developmental Disorders, 45,* 4140–4146. https://doi.org/10.1007/s10803-015-2528-0

Bergen, D., & Fromberg, D. P. (2009). Play and social interaction in middle childhood. *Phi Delta Kappan, 90,* 426–430. https://doi.org/10.1177/003172170909000610

Bond, T., Yan, Z., & Heene, M. (2020). *Applying the Rasch model* (4th ed.). Routledge.

Borelli, J. L., Hong, K., Rasmussen, H. F., & Smiley, P. A. (2017). Reflective functioning, physiological reactivity, and overcontrol in mothers: Links with school-aged children's reflective functioning. *Developmental Psychology, 53,* 1680–1693. https://doi.org/10.1037/dev00 00371

Bristow, S., & Atkinson, C. (2020). Child-led research investigating social, emotional and mental health and wellbeing aspects of playtime. *Educational and Child Psychology, 37,* 115–131.

Brock, R. L., Ramsdell, E. L., Franz, M. R., & Volk, S. (2020). Validation of a behavioral coding system for measuring mutually responsive orientation in intimate relationships. *Psychological Assessment, 32,* 713–725. https://doi.org/10.1037/pas0000826

Bronfenbrenner, U. (1983). The context of development and the development of context. In R. M. Lerner (Ed.), *Developmental psychology: Historical and philosophical perspectives* (pp. 147–184). Erlbaum.

Bundy, A. C., & Du Toit, S. H. J. (2014). Play and leisure. In B. A. B. Schell, G. Gillen, & M. E. Scaffa (Eds.), *Willard & Spackman's occupational therapy* (13th ed., pp. 805–823). Lippincott Williams & Wilkins.

Bundy, A., Wyver, S., Beetham, K. S., Ragen, J., Naughton, G., Tranter, P., . . . Sterman, J. (2015). The Sydney playground project—Levelling the playing field: A cluster trial of a primary school-based intervention aiming to promote manageable risk-taking in children with disability. *BMC Public Health, 15,* 1125. http://doi.org/10.1186/s12889-01502452-4

Butcher, R. L., & Gersch, I. S. (2014). Parental experiences of the "Time Together" home visiting intervention: An attachment theory perspective. *Educational Psychology in Practice, 30,* 1–18. https://doi.org/10.1080/02667363.2013.867254

Cabrera, N. J., Fitzgerald, H. E., Bradley, R. H., & Roggman, L. (2014). The ecology of father–child relationships: An expanded model. *Journal of Family Theory and Review, 6,* 336–354. https://doi.org/10.1111/jftr.12054

Cabrera, N. J., & Roggman, L. (2017). Father play: Is it special? *Infant Mental Health Journal, 38,* 706–708.

Case-Smith, J., & Kuhaneck, H. M. (2008). Play preferences of typically developing children and children with developmental delays between ages 3 and 7 years. *OTJR: Occupation, Participation and Health, 28,* 19–29. https://doi.org/10.3928/15394492-20080101-01

Childress, D. C. (2010). Play behaviors of parents and their young children with disabilities. *Topics in Early Childhood Special Education, 29,* 112–120. https://doi.org/10.1177%2F0271121410390526

Corder, K., Sharp, S. J., Atkin, A. J., Griffin, S. J., Jones, A. P., Ekelund, U., & van Sluijs, E. M. F. (2013). Change in objectively measured physical activity during the transition to adolescence. *British Journal of Sports Medicine, 49,* 730–736. https://doi.org/10.1136/bjsports-2013-093190

De Falco, S., Esposito, G., Venuti, P., & Bomstein, M. H. (2010). Mothers and fathers at play with their children with Down syndrome: Influence on child exploratory and symbolic activity. *Journal of Applied Research in Intellectual Disabilities, 23,* 579–605.

Desmarais, S. (2006). A space to float with someone: Recovering play as a field of repair in work with parents of late-adopted children. *Journal of Child Psychotherapy, 32,* 349–364. https://doi.org/10.1080/00754170600996879

Ebrahim, C., Steen, R. L., & Paradise, L. (2012). Overcoming school counselors' barriers to play therapy. *International Journal of Play Therapy, 21*(4), 202–214.

Every Student Succeeds Act, Pub. L. 114-195, 129 Stat. 1802. (2015).

Fabrizi, S. E., Ito, M. A., & Winston, K. (2016). Effect of occupational therapy-led playgroups in early intervention on child playfulness and caregiver responsiveness: A repeated-measures design. *American Journal of Occupational Therapy, 70,* 700220020. https://doi.org/10.5014/ajot.2016.017012

Feldman, R., & Eidelman, A. I. (2005). Does a triplet birth pose a special risk for infant development? Assessing cognitive development in relation to intrauterine growth and mother–infant interaction across the first 2 years. *Pediatrics, 115,* 443–452. http://dx.doi.org/10.1542/peds.2004-1137

Feldman, R., Keren, M., Gross-Rozval, O., & Tyano, S. (2004). Mother–child touch patterns in infant feeding disorders: Relation to maternal, child, and environmental factors. *Journal of the American Academy of Child and Adolescent Psychiatry, 43,* 1089–1097. https://doi.org/10.1097/01.chi.0000132810.98922.83

Feldman, R., & Klein, P. S. (2003). Toddlers' self-regulated compliance to mothers, caregivers, and fathers: Implications for theories of socialization. *Developmental Psychology, 39,* 680–692. https://doi.org/10.1037/0012-1649.39.4.680

Flanders, J. L., Leo, V., Paquette, D., Pihl, R. O., & Séguin, J. R. (2009). Rough-and-tumble play and the regulation of aggression: An observational study of father–child play dyads. *Aggressive Behavior, 35,* 285–295. https://doi.org/10.1002/ab.20309

Flasch, P., Taylor, D., Clauber, R. N., & Robinson III, E. (2017). Examining students' self-perceived competence and comfort in an experiential play therapy counseling course: A single group pretest-posttest investigation. *International Journal for the Scholarship of Teaching and Learning, 11*(1), 10.

Fonagy, P., & Target, M. (1998). Mentalization and the changing aims of child psychoanalysis. *Psychoanalytic Dialogues, 8,* 87–114. https://doi.org/10.1080/10481889809539235

Frolek Clark, G., & Ponsolle-Mays, M. (2019). The *OTPF–3*: Communicating occupational therapy in schools. In G. Frolek Clark, J. E. Rioux, & B. E. Chandler (Eds.), *Best practices for occupational therapy in schools* (2nd ed.). AOTA Press.

Fujiwara, K., & Daibo, I. (2014). The extraction of nonverbal behaviors: Using video images and speech-signal analysis in dyadic conversation. *Journal of Nonverbal Behavior, 38,* 377–388. https://doi.org/10.1007/s10919-014-0183-3

Gale, E., & Schick, B. (2008). Symbol-infused joint attention and language use in mothers with deaf and hearing toddlers. *American Annals of the Deaf, 153,* 484–503. http://www.jstor.org/stable/26234559

Garfinkel, M., & Minard, C. (2021). Supporting occupational balance in children using everyday technologies: The distinct value of occupational therapy. *SIS Quarterly Practice Connections, 6*(1), 5–7.

Gordon, G. (2014). Well played: The origins and future of playfulness. *American Journal of Play, 6,* 234–266.

Graber, K. M., Byrne, E. M., Goodacre, E. J., Kirby, N., Kulkarni, K., O'Farrelly, C., & Ramchandani, P. G. (2021). A rapid review of the impact of quarantine and restricted environments on children's play and the role of play in children's health. *Child: Care, Health and Development, 47,* 143–153. https://doi.org/10.1111/cch.12832

Graham, N. E., Truman, J., & Holgate, H. (2015). Parents' understanding of play for children with cerebral palsy. *American Journal of Occupational Therapy, 69,* 6903220050. https://doi.org/10.5014/ajot.2015.015263

Gridley, N., Bywater, T. J., & Hutchings, J. M. (2018). Comparing live and video observation to assess early parent–child interactions in the home. *Journal of Child and Family Studies, 27,* 1818–1829. https://doi.org/10.1007/s10826-018-1039-y

Guitard, P., Ferland, F., & Dutil, E. (2005). Toward a better understanding of playfulness in adults. *OTJR: Occupation, Participation and Health, 25,* 9–22. https://doi.org/10.1177/153944920502500103

Harvey, E. A., Friedman-Weieneth, J. L., Miner, A. L., Bartolomei, R. J., Youngwirth, S. D., Hashim, R. L., & Arnold, D. H. (2009). The role of ethnicity in observers' ratings of mother–child behavior. *Developmental Psychology, 45,* 1497–1508. https://doi.org/10.1037/a0017200

Hess, L. M., & Bundy, A. C. (2003). The association between playfulness and coping in adolescents. *Physical and Occupational Therapy in Pediatrics, 23,* 5–17. https://doi.org/10.1080/j006v23n02_02

Howard, J., Miles, G. E., Rees-Davies, L., & Bertenshaw, E. J. (2017). Play in middle childhood: Everyday play behaviour and associated emotions. *Children and Society, 31,* 378–389. https://doi.org/10.1111/chso.12208

Hwang, H. G., & Markson, L. (2020). The development of social exclusion detection in early childhood: Awareness of social exclusion does not always align with social preferences. *Journal of Cognition and Development, 21,* 166–190. https://doi.org/10.1080/15248372.2019.1706521

Imms, C., Froude, E., Adair, B., & Shields, N. (2016). A descriptive study of the participation of children and adolescents in activities outside school. *BMC Pediatrics, 16,* 84. https://doi.org/10.1186/s12887-016-0623-9

Individuals With Disabilities Education Improvement Act of 2004, Pub. L. 108-446, 20 U.S.C. § 1400 *et seq.*

Jago, R., Salway, R., Lawlor, D. A., Emm-Collison, L., Heron, J., Thompson, J. L., & Sebire, S. J. (2018). Profiles of children's physical activity and sedentary behaviour between age 6 and 9: A latent profile and transition analysis. *International Journal of Behavioral Nutrition and Physical Activity, 15*(1), 103. https://doi.org/10.1186/s12966-018-0735-8

John, A., Halliburton, A., & Humphrey, J. (2013). Child–mother and child–father play interaction patterns with preschoolers. *Early Child Development and Care, 183,* 483–497. https://doi.org/10.1080/03004430.2012.711595

Jones, J., & Mosher, W. D. (2013). Fathers' involvement with their children: United States, 2006–2010. *National Health Statistics Reports, 71,* 1–21. https://www.cdc.gov/nchs/data/nhsr/nhsr071.pdf

Keren, M., Feldman, R., Namdari-Weinbaum, I., Spitzer, S., & Tyano, S. (2005). Relations between parents' interactive style in dyadic and triadic play and toddlers' symbolic capacity. *American Journal of Orthopsychiatry, 75,* 599–607. https://doi.org/10.1037/0002-9432.75.4.599

Knox, S. (2008). Development and current use of the Knox Preschool Play Scale. In L. D. Parham & L. S. Fazio (Eds.), *Play in occupational therapy for children* (2nd ed., pp. 35–51). Mosby.

Lam, C. B., & McHale, S. M. (2015). Developmental patterns and parental correlates of youth leisure-time physical activity. *Journal of Family Psychology, 29,* 100–107. https://doi.org/10.1037/fam0000049

Landreth, G. L. (2012). *Play therapy: The art of relationship* (3rd ed.). Routledge/Taylor & Francis.

Laverdure, P., & Beisbier, S. (2021). Occupation- and activity-based interventions to improve performance of activities of daily living, play, and leisure for children and youth ages 5 to 21: A systematic review. *American Journal of Occupational Therapy, 75,* 7501205050. https://doi.org/10.5014/ajot.2021.039560

Lifter, K., Foster-Sanda, S., Arzamarski, C., Briesch, J., & Mcclure, E. (2011). Overview of Play. *Infants and Young Children, 24,* 225–245. https://doi.org/10.1097/iyc.0b013e31821e995c

Lin, Y. W., & Bratton, S. C. (2015). A meta-analytic review of child-centered play therapy approaches. *Journal of Counseling and Development, 93,* 45–58. https://doi.org/10.1002/j.1556-6676.2015. 00180.x

Linacre, J. M. (2022). *Winsteps® Rasch measurement computer program* (Version 5.4). Winsteps.com

Lindsey, E. W., & Mize, J. (2000). Parent–child physical and pretense play: Links to children's social competence. *Merrill-Palmer Quarterly, 46,* 565–588. https://www.jstor.org/stable/23092565

Magnuson, C. D., & Barnett, L. A. (2013). The playful advantage: How playfulness enhances coping with stress. *Leisure Sciences, 35,* 129–144. https://doi.org/10.1080/01490400.2013.761905

Männikkö, N., Ruotsalainen, H., Miettunen, J., Marttila-Tornio, K., & Kääriäinen, M. (2020). Parental socioeconomic status, adoe lescents' screen time and sports participation through externalizing and internalizing characteristics. *Heliyon, 6*(2), e03415. https://doi.org/10.1016/j.heliyon.2020.e03415

McNeil, G. D., & Repetti, R. L. (2021). Everyday emotions: Naturalistic observation of specific positive emotions in daily family life. *Journal of Family Psychology, 35,* 172–181. https://doi.org/10.1037/fam0000655

Mertol-Ilgar, S., & Cigdem-Karakurt, C. (2018). An investigation of the effect of preschool children's computer game playing on their development and behavior through the lens of Turkish mothers. *Universal Journal of Educational Research, 6,* 2855–2863. https://doi.org/10.13189/ujer.2018.061220

Oberle, E., Ji, X. R., Guhn, M., Schonert-Reichl, K. A., & Gadermann, A. M. (2019). Benefits of extracurricular participation in early adolescence: Associations with peer belonging and mental health. *Journal of Youth and Adolescence, 48,* 2255–2270. https://doi.org/10.1007/s10964-019-01110-2

Oren, A. (2008). The use of board games in child psychotherapy. *Journal of Child Psychotherapy, 34,* 364–383. https://doi.org/10.1080/00754170802472893

Parham, L. D., & Primeau, L. A. (2008). Play and occupational therapy. In L. D. Parham & L. S. Fazio (Eds.), *Play in occupational therapy for children* (2nd ed., pp. 2–21). Mosby.

Pascal, C., & Bertram, T. (2021). What do young children have to say? Recognizing their voices, wisdom, agency and need for companionship during the COVID pandemic. *European Early Childhood Education Research Journal, 29,* 21–34. https://doi.org/10.1080/1350293X.2021.1872676

Pereira, J., & Smith-Adcock, S. (2013). An evaluation of a child-centered play therapy workshop for school counselors. *International Journal of Play Therapy, 22,* 129–142.

Pierucci, J. M., Barber, A. B., Gilpin, A. T., Crisler, M. E., & Klinger, L. G. (2015). Play assessments and developmental skills in young children with autism spectrum disorders. *Focus on Autism and Other Developmental Disabilities, 30*(1), 35–43. https://doi.org/10.1177/1088357614539837

Pickens, N. D., & Pizur-Barnekow, K. (2009). Co-occupational: Extending the dialogue. *Journal of Occupational Science, 16,* 151–156. https://doi.org/10.1080/14427591.2009.9686656

Pierce, D. (2009). Co-occupation: The challenges of defining concepts original to occupational science. *Journal of Occupational Science, 16,* 203–207. https://doi.org/10.1080/14427591.2009.9686663

Pierce, D. E. (2014). *Occupational science for occupational therapy.* SLACK.

Pizur-Barnekow, K., Kamp, K., & Cashin, S. (2014). An investigation of maternal play styles during the co-occupation of maternal-infant play. *Journal of Occupational Science, 21,* 202–209. https://doi.org/10.1080/14427591.2012.724379

Pontes, T. B., Silva, B. M., Sousa, J. G., Queiroz De Almeida, P. H. T., Davis, J. A., & Polatajko, H. J. (2016). Measuring children activity repertoire: Is the Paediatric Activity Card Sort a good tool for Brazilian therapists? *Cadernos Braisleiros de Terapia Ocupacional, 24,* 435–445. https://doi.org/10.4322/0104-4931.CTOAO0754

Price, P., & Miner Stephenson, S. (2009). Learning to promote occupational development through co-occupation. *Journal of Occupational Science, 16,* 180–186. https://doi.org/10.1080/14427591.2009.9686660

Proyer, R. T. (2012a). Development and initial assessment of a short measure for adult playfulness: The SMAP. *Personality and Individual Differences, 53*(8), 989–994. https://doi.org/10.1016/j.paid.2012.07.018

Proyer, R. T. (2012b). Examining playfulness in adults: Testing its correlates with personality, positive psychological functioning, goal aspirations, and multi-methodically assessed ingenuity. *Psychological Test and Assessment Modeling, 54,* 103–127.

Proyer, R. T. (2012c). A psycho-linguistic study on adult playfulness: Its hierarchical structure and theoretical considerations. *Journal of Adult Development, 19,* 141–149. https://doi.org/10.1007/s10804-012-9141-7

Ray, D. C., Armstrong, S. A., Balkin, R. S., & Jayne, K. M. (2015). Child-centered play therapy in schools: Review and meta-analysis. *Psychology in the Schools, 52,* 107–123. https://doi.org/10.1002/pits.21798

Rehabilitation Act of 1973, Pub. L. 93-112, 29 U.S.C. §§ 701–796l.

Román-Oyola, R., Bundy, A., Castro, E., Castrillo, O., Morel, K. Y., Molina-Martinez, A., . . . Rosado-Torres, D. (2022). Play and mothers' relationships with children in the context of breast cancer. *OTJR: Occupation, Participation and Health, 43,* 43–51. https://doi.org/10.1177/15394492221093996

Sá, C., Pombo, A., Luz, C., Rodrigues, L. P., & Cordovil, R. (2020). COVID-19 social isolation in Brazil: Effects on the physical activity routine of families with children. *Pediatria de Sao Paulo, 39,* e2020159. https://doi.org/10.1590/1984-0462/2021/39/2020159

Sanches-Ferreira, M., Alves, S., Silveira-Maia, M., Gomes, M., & Santos, B. (2019). Participation in leisure activities as an indicator of inclusion: A comparison between children with and without disabilities in Portugal. *European Journal of Educational Research, 8,* 221–232. https://doi.org/10.12973/eu-jer.8.1.221

Saunders, I., Sayer, M., & Goodale, A. (1999). The relationship between playfulness and coping in preschool children: A pilot study. *American Journal of Occupational Therapy, 53,* 221–226. https://doi.org/10.5014/ajot.53.2.221

Schneiderman, I., Kanat-Maymon, Y., Zagoory-Sharon, O., & Feldman, R. (2014). Mutual influences between partners' hormones shape conflict dialog and relationship duration at the initiation of romantic love. *Social Neuroscience, 9,* 337–351. https://doi.org/10.1080/17470919.2014.893925

Scoggin, A. (1999). Caregiving as an occupation: Developmental intervention for a group of hospitalized Peruvian children. *Journal of Occupational Science, 6,* 34–41. https://doi.org/10.1080/14427591.1999.9686449

Sethi, C. (2020). Mothering as a relational role: Re-evaluating everyday parenting occupations. *Journal of Occupational Science, 27,* 158–169. https://doi.org/10.1080/14427591.2019.1666423

Shai, D., & Belsky, J. (2011). When words just won't do: Introducing parental embodied mentalizing. *Child Development Perspectives, 5,* 173–180. https://doi.org/10.1111/j.1750-8606.2011.00181.x

Shaver, P. R., Mikulincer, M., & Shemesh-Iron, M. (2010). A behavioral systems perspective on prosocial behavior. In M. Mikulincer & P. R. Shaver (Eds.), *Prosocial motives, emotions, and behavior: The better angels of our nature* (pp. 72–91). American Psychological Association.

Shen, X. S., Chick, G., & Zinn, H. (2014). Validating the Adult Playfulness Trait Scale (APTS): An examination of personality, nomological network of playfulness. *American Journal of Play, 6,* 345–369.

Shepherd, J., Hanft, B., & Read, J. S. (2019). Best practices in collaborating on school and community teams. In G. Frolek Clark, J. E. Rioux, & B. E. Chandler (Eds.), *Best practices for occupational therapy in schools* (2nd ed., pp. 93–100). AOTA Press.

Shin, S. M., & Gonzalez, J. (2018). A child-centered play therapy workshop for professional elementary school counselors: An exploratory study. *International Journal of Play Therapy, 27,* 134–145. https://doi.org/10.1037/pla0000072

Skard, G. & Bundy, A. C. (2008). Test of Playfulness. In L. D. Parham & L. S. Fazio (Eds.), *Play in occupational therapy for children* (2nd ed., pp. 71–93). Mosby.

Slade, A. (2007). Reflective parenting programs: Theory and development. *Psychoanalytic Inquiry, 26,* 640–657. https://doi.org/10.1080/07351690701310698

Sparrman, A. (2005). Video recording as interaction: Participant observation of children's everyday life. *Qualitative Research in Psychology, 2,* 241–255. https://doi.org/10.1191/1478088705qp041oa

Sterman, J., Villeneuve, M., Bundy, A., & Wyver, S. (2020). School playground intervention for children with disabilities creates play capabilities and shifts adult perspectives. *American Journal of Occupational Therapy, 74*(4, Suppl. 1), 7411515445. https://doi.org/10.5014/ajot.2020.74S1-PO8122

StGeorge, J., Fletcher, R., Freeman, E., Paquette, D., & Dumont, C. (2015). Father–child interactions and children's risk of injury. *Early Child Development and Care, 185,* 1409–1421. https://doi.org/10.1080/03004430.2014.1000888

Thelen, E., Corbetta, D., Kamm, K., Spencer, J. P., Schneider, K., & Zernicke, R. F. (1993). The transition to reaching: Mapping intention and intrinsic dynamics. *Child Development*, 64, 1058–1098.

Trapnell, P. D., & Campbell, J. D. (1999). Private self-consciousness and the five-factor model of personality: Distinguishing rumination from reflection. *Journal of Personality and Social Psychology, 76,* 284–304. https://doi.org/10.1037/0022-3514.76.2.284

UNICEF. (n.d.). *Convention on the Rights of the Child.* https://www.unicef.org/child-rights-convention/convention-text#

United Nations Convention on the Rights of the Child. (1989). *United Nations Convention on the Rights of the Child.* Geneva: United Nations.

U.S. Department of Health and Human Services. (2006). *Your rights under Section 504 of the Rehabilitation Act.* https://www.hhs.gov/sites/default/files/ocr/civilrights/resources/factsheets/504.pdf#:~:text=Section%20504%20protects%20qualified%20individuals%20with%20disabilities.%20Under,diabetes%2C%20drug%20addiction%2C%20heart%20disease%2C%20and%20mental%20illness

Waldman-Levi, A. (2021). Differences in how mothers and fathers support children playfulness. *Journal of Infant and Child Development, 30,* e2257. https://doi.org/10.1002/icd.2257

Waldman-Levi, A. (2022). Parent-child play and attachment. In H. Miller Kuhaneck & S. L. Spitzer (Eds.), *Making play just right: Activity analysis, creativity, and playfulness in pediatric occupational therapy* (2nd ed., pp. 295–319). Jones & Bartlett Learning.

Waldman-Levi, A., & Bundy, A. (2016). A glimpse into co-occupations: Parent/Caregiver's Support of Young Children's Playfulness Scale. *Occupational Therapy in Mental Health, 32,* 217–227. https://doi.org/10.1080/0164212X.2015.1116420

Waldman-Levi, A., Bundy, A., & Shai, D. (2022). Playfulness development and cognitive capacity among typically developing children: A longitudinal study. *American Journal of Occupational Therapy, 76,* 7605205020. https://doi.org/10.5014/ajot.2022.049120

Waldman-Levi, A., Cope, A., & Olson, L. (2022). Understanding father–child joint play experience using a convergent mixed-methods design. *American Journal of Occupational Therapy, 76,* 7605205070. https://doi.org/10.5014/ajot.2022.046573

Waldman-Levi, A., Finzi-Dottan, R., & Cope, A. (2019). Mother-child joint play: The role of maternal caregiving and reflective function. *Journal of Child Family Studies,* 29, 94–104. https://doi.org/10.1007/s10826-019-01638-8

Waldman-Levi, A., Grinion, S., & Olson, L. (2019). Effects of maternal views and support on childhood development through joint play. *Open Journal of Occupational Therapy, 7*(4), 1–21. https://doi.org/10.15453/2168-6408.1613

Waldman-Levi, A., Olson, L., Sheills, M., Melendez-Horvath, M., Corbett, K., & Bundy, A. (2017, March 30–April 2). *Co-occupations: Feasibility of a comprehensive in-depth assessment procedure* [Poster]. American Occupational Therapy Association Annual Conference & Expo, Philadelphia.

Waldman-Levi, A., & Weintraub, N. (2009). Occupational therapy intervention for mothers and their children who were victims of domestic violence. *Israeli Journal of Occupational Therapy, 18,* 97–116.

Waldman-Levi, A., & Weintraub, N. (2015). Efficacy of a crisis intervention for improving mother–child interaction and the children's play functions. *American Journal of Occupational Therapy, 69,* 6901220020. https://doi.org/10.5014/ajot.2015.013375

Wang, Y. Z., Wiley, A. R., & Zhou, X. (2007). The effect of different cultural lenses on reliability and validity in observational data: The example of Chinese immigrant parent–toddler dinner interactions. *Social Development, 16,* 777–799. https://doi.org/10.1111/j.1467-9507.2007.00407.x

Whitcomb, D. A. (2012). Attachment, occupation, and identity: Considerations in infancy. *Journal of Occupational Science, 19,* 271–282. https://doi.org/10.1080/14427591.2011.634762

Winnicott, D. W. (1999). *The child, the family and the outside world.* Sifriat Poalim Publishing.

Wright, M. (2021). *How every child can thrive by five* [Video]. TED Conferences. https://www.ted.com/talks/molly_wright_how_every_child_can_thrive_by_five/transcript?language=en

Zahl, T., Steinsbekk, S., & Wichstrøm, L. (2017). Physical activity, sedentary behavior, and symptoms of major depression in middle childhood. *Pediatrics, 139*(2), e20161711. https://doi.org/10.1542/peds.2016-1711

Appendixes

APPENDIX A. Scoring Form

Dyad (#): **Age:** **Rater:** **In** **Out** **Video** **Live** **(Circle)**		**Scale** **NA = not applicable** **0 = low** **1 = mild** **2 = moderate** **3 = high**
Items	**Score**	**Comments**
1. Parent/caregiver is *actively supporting* the child's engagement in free play.		
2. Parent/caregiver supports the child's engagement in the activity *for the process* rather than primarily for the end product (building, assembling, and "getting the job done").		
3. Parent/caregiver *helps* the child *overcome barriers or obstacles* to persist with the activity.		
4. Parent/caregiver demonstrates *positive affect* during play.		
5. Parent/caregiver *supports* the child in *decision making*.		
6. Parent/caregiver provides *a sense of safety* during play, so the child will feel sufficiently safe (emotionally and physically) to keep playing (e.g., selecting toys, coming up with ideas, making modifications, feeling safe to make choices or move around).		
7. Parent/caregiver *supports* the child's *modifications* or their need to *modify* the activity to maintain the challenge or make it more fun.		
8. Parent/caregiver *supports the child in interacting with objects* during play.		
9. Parent/caregiver *supports* the child's *transition* from one activity to the other when the first no longer evolves or suits the child preferences or needs or supports the child to remain with an activity that is meeting the child's needs.		
10. Parent/caregiver *supports* the child's *negotiations* to have their desires met in a suitable, respectful, and age-appropriate manner.		
11. Parent/caregiver *supports* the child's needs in *social play*.		
12. Parent/caregiver *supports* the child's engagement in playful *mischief, clowning*, or *joking*, or the parent/caregiver incorporates *mischief, clowning, or joking* during play.		

(Continued)

APPENDIX A. Scoring Form *(Cont.)*

Items	**Score**	**Comments**
13. Parent/caregiver *supports* the child's *pretending* (to be someone else; to do something else; that an object is something else; that something else is happening). Parent/caregiver may enter into the pretend play as well.		
14. Parent/caregiver *supports* or encourages the child to *incorporate* objects or other people into play in *unconventional or variable* ways.		
15. Parent/caregiver adheres to *consistent, reasonable, and clear boundaries or rules.* Rules do not change unexpectedly.		
16. Parent/caregiver *verbally praises* the child for a desired and appropriate behavior during play interactions.		
Average score	**Sum of column scores/16 or number of items scored, excluding items scored NA**	

Appendix B. Key Form

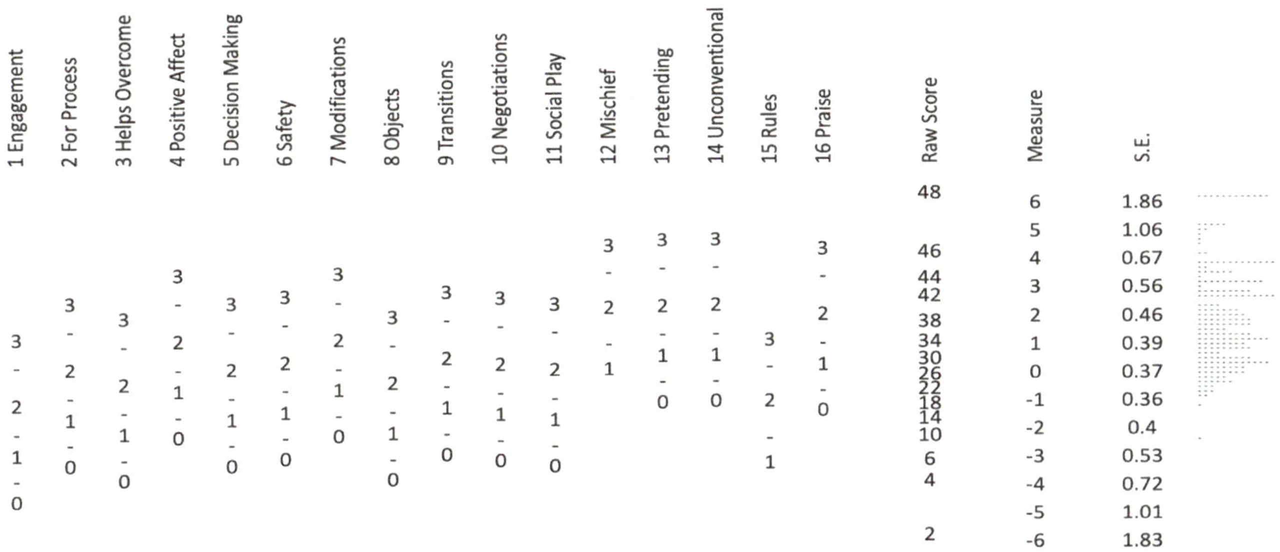